KW-338-668

Crime in Europe

Edited by
Frances Heidensohn
and
Martin Farrell

ROUTLEDGE
London and New York

For Klaus and Korinna

First published in 1991
by Routledge
11 New Fetter Lane, London EC4P 4EE

First published in paperback in 1993

Simultaneously published in the USA and Canada
by Routledge
29 West 35th Street, New York, NY 10001

© 1991 Frances Heidensohn and Martin Farrell; additional material
© 1993 Frances Heidensohn and Martin Farrell

Typeset in Baskerville by LaserScript, Mitcham, Surrey
Printed and bound in Great Britain by
Mackays of Chatham PLC, Kent

All rights reserved. No part of this book may be reprinted or reproduced or utilized in any form or by any electronic, mechanical, or other means, now known or hereafter invented, including photocopying and recording, or in any information storage or retrieval system, without permission in writing from the publishers.

British Library Cataloguing in Publication Data
Crime in Europe.
1. Western Europe. Crimes. Prevention
I. Heidensohn, Frances II. Farrell, Martin *1950*
364.4094

Library of Congress Cataloging in Publication Data
Crime in Europe/edited by Frances Heidensohn and Martin Farrell.
p. cm.
Papers originally presented at a conference organized by the Institute for the Study and Treatment of Delinquency, held at the University of York, in September 1988.
Includes bibliographical references.
1. Crime – Europe – Congresses. 2. Crime prevention – Europe – Congresses. 3. Criminology – Europe – Congresses. I. Heidensohn, Frances. II. Farrell, Martin, 1950–. III. Institute for the Study and Treatment of Delinquency (Great Britain)
HV6938.5.C75 1990 90-8423
364.94–dc20 CIP

ISBN 0-415-05072-3 (hbk)
0-415-09649-9 (pbk)

Crime in Europe

SEVEN DAY LOAN
This book is to be returned on
or before the date stamped below

17 NOV 2000
23.11.00
17 JAN 2001
22 OCT 2001
26 NOV 2001
17 JAN 2003
– 3 FEB 2003
– 2 JUN 2003
13 JAN 2004

UNIVERSITY OF PLYMOUTH
PLYMOUTH LIBRARY
Tel: (01752) 232323
This book is subject to recall if required by another reader
Books may be renewed by phone
CHARGES WILL BE MADE FOR OVERDUE BOOKS

While some European nations share similar crime rates and trends, many differ widely in their approach to criminal justice. And, as Europe's internal frontiers give way to the 'single market', issues such as the control of terrorists, international fraud and drug trafficking take on significant dimensions. This is the first book to address these issues and attempt a comparative criminology for Europe.

The contributions cover a range of subjects including crime prevention, [illegible] the relationship of ethnic minorities to crime and the police, corporate crime, and accountability in the prison system.

30

90 0725301 6

Contents

UNIVERSITY OF PLYMOUTH
LIBRARY SERVICES
Item No. 900138933X
Class No. 364.94 CRI
Contl No. 0415050723

Illustrations

FIGURES

TABLES

Contributors

Hans-Jörg Albrecht is research fellow at the Max-Planck-Institute for Foreign and International Criminal Law in Freiburg, Federal Republic of Germany.

Ewa Bienkowska is Assistant Professor at the Institute of State and Law, Polish Academy of Sciences, Warsaw, Poland.

Jan van Dijk is Director of the Crime Prevention Department at the Ministry of Justice, The Hague, the Netherlands.

Nick Dorn is Development Director of the Institute for the Study of Drug Dependence (ISDD), London, England.

Martin Farrell was Director of the Institute for the Study and Treatment of Delinquency (ISTD), London, and is now at the British Red Cross, London, England.

Cyrille Fijnaut is Professor of Criminology and Criminal Law at the Catholic University of Leuven, Belgium.

Frances Heidensohn is Reader in the Social Policy and Politics Department, Goldsmiths' College, University of London, England.

Michael Levi is Professor in Criminology in the University of Wales.

Marie-Pierre de Liège is Inspecteur des Services Judiciares (Inspector of Judicial Services), Ministry of Justice, Paris.

Christa Pelikan is Research Officer at the Institute of the Sociology of Law and Crime in Vienna, Austria.

Joanna Shapland is Lecturer in Law at the Department of Law, University of Sheffield, England.

Nigel South is Lecturer in Sociology at the University of Essex, England.

Jon Vagg is Lecturer in Sociology at the University of Hong Kong.

Preface and acknowledgements

These papers were originally given at the Institute for the Study and Treatment of Delinquency's conference entitled 'Crime in Europe', held at the University of York in September 1988. Discussions at the conference, and in other settings, revealed the importance of this topic and of the many issues raised in connection with it. It was also clear that relatively little writing was available which addressed these issues. This collection is therefore being published as an initial step in focusing the developing interest in crime in Europe and in a European approach to crime. The importance of this selection lies both in the individual subjects covered as well as their presentation together: they demonstrate range and variety as well as several major themes and an agenda for future work.

While the conference marked a significant step in a new direction for the Institute, it was also in part a return to its origins. The ISTD was founded in 1931 under strong European influences, notably from the (then) innovatory treatment of offenders by psychotherapy. Since the 1930s, the Institute's programme has developed to include a much wider range of activities, including the *British Journal of Criminology* (Europe's leading academic journal in the field), a series of visits to European countries to study their criminal justice systems and further conferences since the one recorded here. We are conscious, then, of both tradition and change in our own Institute and its role in presenting and studying the new crime agenda in Europe.

In presenting the papers collected here, we are very conscious that they are only a sample of those given at the conference. This selection does, we believe, convey both the range of issues to be addressed in studying crime in Europe and the insights to be gained from comparative study. Our hope is that this volume will stimulate discussion, lead to further research and conferences and raise the profile of one of the most important social problems faced by Europe, east and west, as the twentieth century draws to a close.

Mounting a major international conference and then editing some of its papers for publication is a formidable task. To complete it we have had to call on the help and advice of many people. We should particularly like to thank our fellow members of the Waldorf Group – Jean Taylor, Keith Cockman and John Freeman – who planned the conference with us. At ISTD, Douglas Acres, the Chairman of the Education Committee, gave invaluable support, as did Irene Frost and Joan Worth in producing this volume. Talia Rodgers has given us enthusiastic editorial advice and Joanna Shapland commented most helpfully on an earlier draft. Key contributions at the conference on which we have drawn in compiling this selection came from Hans-Jürgen Bartsch, Jillian Becker, John Bell, Simon Buxton, Geoffrey Cartledge, David Downes, David Faulkner, Henri Giller, John Graham, Chris Holtom and Christina Steen-Sundberg.

The European Cultural Foundation provided funding for the conference and we gratefully acknowledge their generosity. Frances Heidensohn was granted sabbatical leave in the academic year 1987–8 by Goldsmiths' College and this enabled her to spend some time on preparing material in this publication.

We are both fortunate in having strong personal as well as criminological links to Europe. Editing *Crime in Europe* has helped us to learn a great deal about European co-operation. We trust that all those close to us, because they share our interest and enthusiasm, have felt that this has been a worthwhile project and one to which they have been able to contribute.

We met to plan and edit this book in the Palm Court of the Waldorf Hotel in London; we should like to thank the manager and his staff for their courtesy and patience and to record our appreciation of their incomparable afternoon teas.

Frances Heidensohn
Martin Farrell

Preface to the paperback edition

The publication of *Crime in Europe* in paperback gives us the chance of reviewing its content and messages and seeing how much they need to be updated. This book has certainly been produced during a period of very rapid, and often dramatic, change. The demolition of the Berlin Wall began as we finished the final draft of the manuscript; the Gulf War ended just before its appearance in hardback; former Yugoslavia is in turmoil as this is being written. How far do we need to revise the original content of *Crime in Europe* to reflect these developments?

There are four areas to focus on: some important changes in names, the impact of key social changes, developments in Eastern Europe and Europe-wide policy initiatives.

ALTERED STATES

Two shifts have occurred which have led to a redrawing of the boundaries of various European states named in this book. The reunification of Germany has in practice meant the abolition of the German Democratic Republic, and is the sole instance of refederation in modern Europe. Elsewhere, especially in the East and South the pattern has been one of balkanization, of splitting into smaller independent entities, of which the break up of the former Soviet Union is the most dramatic example. Most cases have been contested and in some, armed conflict has resulted and continues at the time of writing. Hence, we have not attempted to set out a list of such changes, but merely wish to draw the reader's attention to the problem.

MAJOR SOCIAL CHANGES

The topics which are the focus of this book and which are highlighted in the Introduction, such as drugs, terrorism, fraud, racism, have all continued to be highly topical and, if anything, to have increased in importance. The cases of the Bank of Credit and Commerce International, and of the late Robert Maxwell illustrate the problem of modern fraud organisation, while violence against ethnic minorities has been a growing problem in several European countries. We have developed some of the arguments raised here in a later paper which examines the impact of certain social conditions (Heidensohn and Farrell 1991).

It could well be said that the processes of social change have speeded up considerably since the first edition was prepared. However, both the topics selected and the trends discerned have proved robust and we would not wish to alter the overall balance and arguments of the book.

EASTERN EUROPE

The former communist-run states of Eastern Europe have seen the most rapid dramatic changes in their political structures and these have particular significance for criminality. As Chapter 4, 'Crime in Eastern Europe', outlines, publication of data on crime was, before the recent political changes, a very limited exercise. Criminal statistics were often not published at all, or else were accessible only to a select group; judicial figures were compromised still more. Data have now become available from most administrations. Partly as a result of this freer source of information, but also because of a changed climate for the debate and discussion of social problems, there has been a spate of studies and articles on crime and deviant behaviour in the former communist states. Common themes include whether capitalist freedom is criminogenic and the alleged increase of violent offending in these societies. It is clear that, while such work represents major advances, answers to these and other questions remain conjectural and controversial.

POLICY DEVELOPMENTS

In our original introduction we stress that crime was not a topic on the agenda of the European Community. This position has now changed: the EC sponsored a Europe-wide conference at Cambridge in March 1992 and a sponsored forum and database are proposed. Further European initiatives have also developed, including the setting up of Europol, an information-exchange system, and the formalising of *Schengenland*, the frontier-free territory for the main EC countries. The Maastricht Treaty included agreements to pursue closer co-operation on security matters, including especially, the high policing agenda of drugs and terrorism.

While these changes should be noted (and some references are given below) our main purposes in compiling this collection remain; we hope it will encourage awareness and stimulate debate.

Frances Heidensohn
Martin Farrell
September 1992

BIBLIOGRAPHY

Arbeitsbericht zum Fortsetzungsantrag an die Deutsche Forschungs gemeinschaft, Sozialer Umbruch und Kriminalitätsentwicklung auf dem Gebiet der ehemaligen DDR, Berlin, 1992.

Butler, W. E. (1992) 'Crime in the Soviet Union: early glimpses of the true story', *British Journal of Criminology*, 32, 2: 144–59.

Dashkov, G. V. (1992) 'Quantitative and qualitative changes in crime in the USSR', *British Journal of Criminology*, 32, 2: 160–6.

Heidensohn, F. and Farrell, M. (1991) 'Social welfare and social change in Europe' in G. Room (ed.) *Towards a European Welfare State?*, Bristol: SAUS.

McLaughlin, E. (1992) 'The democratic deficit. European union and the accountability of the British police', *British Journal of Criminology*, 32, 4.

UK Offender Employment Alliance (1992) 'Euro crime, Euro solutions', Interim Report, London: Apex Trust.

Part one

Crime and Europe

Chapter one

Introduction

Convergence, diversity and change

Frances Heidensohn

'Europe' and all things European have become matters of increasing importance in the late twentieth century. The Single European Act and the removal of barriers to trade and to labour mobility after 1992 were the first points of focus. Other changes have also, however, had significant impact. The building of the Channel Tunnel between Britain and France was one of these. On a much wider level, the major developments in Eastern Europe, with their profound political, economic and social consequences, affected the whole of Europe, not least in making the *definition* of Europe itself problematic.

In predicting the prospects of the new Europe, however defined, many topics have been addressed, but crime has been included amongst them only quite recently. Clearly barriers are not being removed nor the Channel Tunnel built in order to improve the effectiveness of supranational policing. It is as realisation of the likely effects of these policies has grown that concerns are expressed by the police and other agencies about them.

It can, indeed, be argued that, until the 1980s, crime in Europe was not a conceptual framework which would have had meaning, save for the select participants in the regular Council of Europe Colloquia. By the time of the conference for which these papers were originally written, it had become a recognisable theme for several reasons. First, and most obviously, the political developments in the European Community nations have made it so, and not least because while other social consequences of 1992 and after had been well explored, and were the clear responsibility of designated bodies, those for crime, for policing and criminal justice had not been and were not so clearly defined as Fijnaut and Levi show devastatingly in this volume (Chapters 8 and 12).

In addition to the policy issues thus raised, developments in the study of crime have helped produce a climate more favourable to comparative criminological study. As Shapland shows (Chapter 2), while criminology has developed in distinctive ways in European nations there have been powerful trends towards homogeneity. The growth of victim studies is only one example of what she notes as common needs of consumers and policy-makers in criminal justice. Another influence undoubtedly comes from the growth of comparative studies in welfare and via social policy where theoretical developments are more fully realised. As the links between crime and welfare and social control have become more apparent, so has the need for concepts and frameworks to explain them as is apparent in the sections on France and Austria in this volume (Chapters 9 and 11).

Crime in Europe is thus on policy and intellectual agendas for the 1990s. The purpose of this volume is fourfold. First, the papers here provide background and foreground material on a wide range of items appearing on both agendas: policing, drugs, terrorism and fraud will all be true 'European' issues. Second, a number of major questions are raised and explored here, such as the effects of barrier removal on policing and the possibilities of a Europe-wide force. Such questions cannot be fully answered as yet. Other sections fulfil a third aim and show the scope of systematic comparative study of crime. Finally, throughout the book Europe's diverse criminological heritage summarised by Shapland (Chapter 2) informs the chapters and suggests the scope of future work in this field.

Most of the continental authors are lawyers while the British are social scientists. Shapland notes not only this difference but also that the dominant influences on British criminology in the twentieth century – Grünhut, Mannheim and Radzinowicz – were all European lawyers. (Roger Hood has observed that the historical impact of these influences has tended to be neglected and remain unexplored.) Differences in method and approach follow from the varied discipline perspectives as do matters of concern. The contributions to this book have sufficient linking themes and topics to illustrate a convincing argument not merely for a volume devoted to crime in Europe, but also for the possibilities of a European criminology.

My aims in this introductory chapter are therefore threefold. The first is to set the whole collection in its context as a contribution to developments and discussions in and about late-twentieth-century Europe. Second, I shall highlight the main current themes in the area of crime both generally and as they are illustrated here. Finally I shall outline some of the problems and the policy issues which now feature on the 'Crime in Europe' agenda and are likely to continue to do so.

BACKGROUND: EUROPE, THE MODERN CAREER OF A CONCEPT

The Second World War was very much a European war. At, or within a few years of, its conclusion the nation-states of continental Europe had formed two geo-political groupings round which were a fringe of neutral states. In 1957, six of the countries of the 'West' signed the Treaty of Rome, pledging themselves to remove tariff barriers and form an economic community. Britain joined the European Economic Community in 1973, together with Ireland and Denmark. By 1988 there were twelve member states and others, including possibly former Eastern Bloc countries, are likely to join in the 1990s. For four decades most of Eastern Europe developed on very different social, political and economic lines from the west with planned, command economies, not plural, capitalist ones.

However, rapid and dramatic changes in the USSR and Poland, as well as in other Warsaw Pact countries, reshaped the social and political map of Europe in the late 1980s. 'Europe' not only meant a geographical landmass and its offshore islands, but also suggested the possibility of something much more. The 'core' of the new Europe is formed by the Community States, which should have no internal trade barriers after 1992. As well as economic integration, wider unification especially of certain key social policies is also being proposed and debated.

Beyond the European Community (EC) nations lie the non-aligned states, mostly with highly sophisticated political and economic systems and notably comprehensive welfare. While these two groupings are certainly likely to be affected by the planned EC changes in the 1990s, it is in and from Eastern Europe that the most notable changes of the decade are likely to come as political icebergs melt like snowballs in the sun. Much has been spoken and written about both the planned and the unplanned changes, which will alter the concept of 'Europe' itself, yet one important issue has received relatively little attention: crime in Europe.

Social Europe for example (the EC's social affairs directorate journal), in its special report on 'The social dimension of the internal market' (Commission of the European Communities 1988), presents detailed material on education, unemployment, migration, wages, etc., but does not mention crime. This is a notable omission for a number of reasons. It is a sociological truism that crime is a social phenomenon and varies with social conditions and economic climates. Indeed, it is clear from several chapters in this volume that there has for some time been concern in several European countries about rising crime rates (Chapters 3, 4, 9 and 11). Some of this concern has been translated into international action where specific wider threats have been identified in terrorism (Chapter 8), drug abuse (Chapter 6) and fraud (Chapter 12). These have been, for the most part, reactive responses to crises.

Yet there has been so far a relatively modest response to the crime possibilities offered by 'Europe' itself. To take only EC nations, for example: can terrorists move as freely as trucks once customs and passport controls are removed? Will there be 'infiltration' as illicit drugs are carried from a relatively open market to a tightly controlled one? How will gun control laws be unified from their present enormous diversity? Many other Europe-wide trends are likely to influence crime patterns in the 1990s, some of them influenced by European policies. Labour mobility shifts not only workers but also patterns of social control and family life. Some of the migrant workers will be skilled, affluent, 'legal' and accepted. Others will be part of a semi-legal underclass, vulnerable to exploitation, even violence (Chapter 7). Some of both groups may be from ethnic minorities whose apparent participation and victimisation rates in relation to crime raise central issues of public policy.

Crime should therefore already be a key issue for all European countries in the 1990s, through the unintended consequences of planned policies in EC countries, major political developments, especially in Eastern Europe which may generate social changes such as migration, new patterns of urbanisation and industrialisation, which are very much linked with trends in crime.

KEY ISSUES

Crime has not yet achieved the same high profile as a European topic as have, for example, wine lakes and butter mountains or the European Monetary System. There have, however, been growing signs of concern from the public and politicians over a number of events. In the late 1980s, for example, the behaviour of English football hooligans at matches abroad, especially after the Heysel disaster, in which thirty-nine people died, caused mounting anger and led to English clubs being banned and to calls for identity cards, passport confiscation and preventive detention (Williams *et al.* 1989). Detention of British subjects in Spanish and Swedish gaols for alleged drug offences focused interest on the different criminal justice systems of other European nations (Alderson 1989). A 'hot pursuit' chase across the German frontier, as well as a series of terrorist incidents made questions about police co-operation and co-ordination highly topical (*Police Review* 1989d).

Alongside popular and media preoccupation with these matters there have been a growing number of conferences and debates which have highlighted issues in several areas (Hood 1989). From the papers delivered at the York conference we have made the following selection which should contribute to understanding, analysis and debate about crime in Europe. Three major themes emerged at the conference and are illustrated in the chapters in this book: convergence, diversity and change. It was also constantly stressed that failure to recognise and confront the effects of these issues could have serious consequences.

Convergence

As van Dijk points out in Chapter 3, crime in Europe appears in some senses to know no frontiers even before these are formally abolished. As he shows, there is remarkable congruence between recorded crime rates in the major west European nations. Bienkowska (Chapter 4) suggests that in the three East European countries she analyses, crime rates are considerably lower than in the west, but that they are highest in the most affluent, the German Democratic Republic. Heidensohn (Chapter 5) shows that female crime rates are relatively low and fairly similar throughout Europe; Albrecht (Chapter 7) finds common patterns in victimisation rates among ethnic minorities in several countries, as well as common misunderstandings about their participation rates and their perceptions. Dorn and South (Chapter 6) note that while illicit drug use was once confined to relatively few parts of Europe, it is now found everywhere. While some of these observations are based on official figures which should be treated carefully, there are clearly enough consistencies to raise interesting questions.

Are there, for example, social influences which spread consistently across the continent and are associated with crime? Is crime indeed a product of affluence, anomie and anti-authoritarianism as van Dijk suggests? What would the consequences be of the growing aspirations of so many Europeans? Or of the 'harmonised' economic future? On the other hand, crime rates in Europe are not consistently correlated with Gross National Product.

Another form of convergence can be found in the Europeanising or internationalising of some forms of criminal activity. While the majority of offences and offenders are still petty and local, some lend themselves to multinational organisation. Levi (Chapter 12) shows how fraudsters move easily from one state to another and increasingly exploit the potential of an open market. Dorn and South outline drug-trafficking trails while Heidensohn points out that prostitution is one of the most established international rackets.

Perhaps one of the most surprising conclusions one can draw from the papers here, as indeed from other symposia (see especially Hood 1989), is that there is considerable congruence in definitions of what constitutes crime problems and issues between different nation-states in Europe. This is not, of course, to say that 'crime' always means the same thing everywhere, or that it can be a meaningful and useful category. Clearly this is a much more complex question. It is, however, worth stressing the impact of three discernible but distinctive trends which appear to have aided this development. First, there is the '*internationalising*' of certain crimes which are not confined to any one nation or even continent: terrorism, drug offences, fraud exemplify this. Second, *common social influences* have rendered much of the capitalist world a 'global village' in another sense, where everyone objects to petty crime, minor incivilities and vandalism and to expensive, and repressive, criminal justice agencies. Finally, there is what we can call the *diffusion of new discovery*, especially of a new crime agenda and of concern for victims of crime. Because of the impact of all these features of the modern world, common definitions of crime as a problem are far more readily understood than either recent criminological orthodoxy or common sense would expect.

While trends and patterns in crime rates across Europe show

either consistency or a tendency to converge, rather less harmony appears in the responses to crime among European nations. Some parallels are manifest. Crime control has become a major issue for most governments as have victim support and policies to deal with fears of crime (van Dijk, de Liège and Pelikan – Chapters 3, 9 and 11). Co-operation between police forces has been increased in response to terrorism, organised crime and drug-trafficking (Fijnaut, Chapter 8). An important external influence has produced some convergence in some areas. US Government policies require its allies to adopt the same approaches to drug use (Dorn and South), control of fraud (Levi), and terrorism (Fijnaut).

Diversity

While some European nations already have common crime patterns or are subject to similar international crime trends, their criminal justice systems and their crime and penal policies differ markedly. Van Dijk shows that it is impossible to predict either overall expenditure on crime control from crime rates, or, more specifically, imprisonment rates. Vagg (Chapter 10) notes diversity in prison regimes, with Britain being more out of step than other nations. Levi finds enormous variation in control of fraud, as do Dorn and South in drugs policies. Fijnaut stresses the enormous variation in policing systems, the hostility between them and the failure of attempts to co-ordinate their efforts. Pelikan's description of a mediation experiment in a country with a written constitution, de Liège's of crime control in a centralised system and Bienkowska's view of Eastern Europe, where crime figures can be state secrets, all illustrate the varied complexity and the range of European crime policies. They also emphasise that there are critical lines which divide Britain, which has no written constitution or Ministry of Justice from other European nations. Again, policing still is a very different concept to many Europeans who have lived under fascist police states (Chapter 3) than it may still be to those who know the Anglo-American idea of police. What is notable about European diversities in responses to crime is that they are largely imposed upon crime patterns which appear consistent or converging.

Change

Throughout the papers in this volume runs a common thread of increasing social changes. From the position of women (Heidensohn) to the greying of the population (van Dijk) and the widespread movement of peoples in search of work or political freedom (Albrecht) present and future Europe is in flux. Crime is always linked to change. Crime rates generally rise in periods of upheaval, though the issue is complex. Certain specific changes in political frontiers and policies post-1992 may well have marked effects on crime rates and several chapters address these questions (Dorn and South, Fijnaut, Levi). What is striking is that relatively little attention has been given to these topics until recently.

It seems unlikely that the colourful diversity of criminal justice systems in Europe will survive harmonisation elsewhere without damage. European court judgments as well as EC directives already affect citizens' lives directly in Britain. Incorporation of the European Convention on Human Rights into English law is a not inconceivable possibility which would have profound consequences. However, while the future may hold promise of growing civil rights, a major paradox of the new, freer, more mobile Europe may be that its growth may be paralleled by pressures for more control: for identity cards, more computers and other hardware, more sophisticated (and secret) police organisation, curbs on football fans and AIDS/HIV carriers, more defensible space and higher levels of private security, more and longer prison sentences. In short while Europe should be more conscious of crime it should not allow its citizens' civil rights to be crushed by that consciousness (Levi, van Dijk).

TOWARDS COMPARATIVE CRIMINOLOGY

It is one purpose of this book to illustrate the scope for the comparative study of crime across Europe. In order to study crime comparatively three conditions need to be met. There must be sources of material and data with which to make comparisons: crime statistics, victim surveys, research studies. Second, translatable concepts have to be available to make possible the collecting, ordering and analysis of such data. Finally, some kind of framework, part universe of discourse, part set of common concerns, must exist.

It is hard as yet to meet all these conditions readily: the USSR began to publish reliable crime statistics only in 1988. There are, however, already existing examples which illustrate some of the fecund potential of such approaches.

The fascinating and complex arguments about the 'dispersal of discipline' thesis in which Foucault's attempt at a vast project on the development of social control in western societies has been used and challenged by a variety of writers is just one example of the possibilities (Foucault 1977; Cohen 1985; Scull 1984; Bottoms 1983; Ashworth 1988; Ignatieff 1978). Another lies in the work of feminist writers who have analysed the nature of formal and informal social control in relation to gender (Heidensohn 1985; Eaton 1986; Smart 1977). This work is well illustrated in Cain's (1989) collection of European studies which show the extent of, and in which she attempts to theorise, the policing and the experiences of young women in modern Europe. Notably, both these projects have produced work at a variety of conceptual levels: in both the role of the state and of penal and criminal justice agencies is theorised and at the same time, detailed empirical case studies published. As yet, other enterprises are still at the stage of beginning to ask interesting questions. How can we, for example, explain differences in penal policies in nations with apparently similar social conditions and crime problems? Downes suggests (1988) that the notable differences between British and Dutch penal policies have several causes, notably the common education and approach of members of the Dutch judicial system as compared with the British and also the 'culture of tolerance' permeating Dutch society which enables people to accept deviance more readily and to be less punitive towards deviants than in Britain.

The contributions in this volume raise many such questions and provide some guidance in reaching the answers.

AN AGENDA FOR CRIME IN EUROPE

Symposia such as the one on which this book is based are important generating sources for new agenda. This one was no exception. From the many topics raised two key areas of criminology and crime policy emerged as most important.

Criminological questions

Research

The chapters in this volume all contribute to the comparative study of crime in Europe. They variously present case studies (Vagg, Pelikan, de Liège), comparative analyses (Vagg, van Dijk, Bienkowska, Heidensohn) or make cross-national comparisons on particular topics (Dorn and South, Levi, Fijnaut). Most comparative work in this field has tended to compare the USA with other countries and has ignored the proximity of European nations. Yet as these chapters illustrate, there is immense scope for comparative work. There are of course problems. A major issue is data (van Dijk, Bienkowska, Heidensohn). Publication and dissemination of research findings are others. Suitable comparative models and theories will also be necessary. It is notable that whereas European theorists once exercised considerable influence (Shapland), now criminologists write in English and their theories are American (Heidensohn).

Crime policy

Crime policy at a European level is no one's business, although the Council of Europe does take an overall interest, it has no actual powers in these matters. Instead national governments and the supranational bodies make policies which affect crime rates and trends with little awareness of their crime-related consequences. There are obvious needs for more and better information on crime and its consequences, for some measures of co-operation and co-ordination (Fijnaut) and also for the wider diffusion of good and successful policies (de Liège, Pelikan). Britain now has the highest imprisonment rate of any European nation; other countries have reduced their prison populations without increasing crime rates (Downes 1988; Graham 1990b). There may be harsh lessons to be learnt as well as positive ones as the failures of Europe-wide police co-ordination suggest (Fijnaut).

In the 1990s Europe will be affected by major trends which are already making crime international. Trade in drugs and in pornographic material already know no frontiers; fraudsters grow yearly more skilful at relocating their enterprises. These factors are not particularly European, but will affect Europe as a whole because in Europe are concentrated many major urban areas and much personal wealth. There will, however, be some distinctively European aspects of crime policy: pressures to standardise and unify within the European Community will affect criminal justice, policing, even penal policy. Labour mobility and attendant social changes will focus attention on such issues as the creation of an 'underclass' (Field 1989) and the marginalisation of some social groups. Political upheavals and nationalist aspirations are likely to bring new protest and perhaps terrorist groups into the political arena. The existence of European justice agencies, however limited their scope, will provide more focus for citizens in search of redress. We face, in short, a future with some Eurocrime and Euroterrorism; whether we shall see Eurocops, Europrisons or Eurojustice is much less clear. The papers in this volume are intended to clarify some of the issues involved.

In introducing his text *Comparative Criminology* in 1965, Hermann Mannheim, a truly European criminologist of his day, suggested

> Criminology, unhampered by the limits of any national legislation, can afford to tackle its problems in a world wide spirit. Actually the opportunity has not always been taken, in part because of language difficulties, in part because of the varying nature of the problems concerned and the existing contrasts in approach and outlook.
>
> (Mannheim 1965: 21)

Mannheim thought at that time that the situation had changed enough to make a true comparative criminology possible. We are sure that it ought to be so now.

The USA is often cited as a model for the future of Europe: a federal nation, diverse yet united. It would be sad if Europe did ever reach the American levels and patterns of crime. Instead it would be more appropriate to beware the many hazards of that model and seek a future where the natural experiments of geographical proximity give scope for comparisons and innovations, but with the possibility of stability as well as change. American enquiry, in short, backed by European tradition. This volume of papers is presented as a contribution to achieving that end.

© 1991 Frances Heidensohn

Chapter two

Criminology in Europe

Joanna Shapland

To describe criminology in Europe is an almost impossible task. The question of 'What is criminology?' has echoed down through the years in each country, fuelled by the constantly reviving debates over the boundaries between criminology and other 'ologies'. They are territorial battles over intellectual spheres of interest, which yet often reflect deeper paradigmatic changes in ideas about the nature of crime and of offending, about their social and individual roots. The question of 'What is criminology?' takes on a more problematic form in the wider terrain of Europe. Though there is no country in which only one model of criminology exists, yet there are still cultural traditions of criminology which render its practice and theoretical enquiry different in the different countries. It is a situation in which it is tempting to offer stereotypes, but one that is changing rapidly, and in which those stereotypes offer too facile and too superficial a solution. This chapter can only be a personal – and very partial and limited – view of some of those traditions.

Perhaps the debates and impermanence of solutions are endemic to the subject and the organisation of the way in which criminologists come to the subject and then develop within it. There are few places and periods that have allowed the permanence of funding and concentration of workers that permit the emergence of strong schools of thought or strong traditions of empirical enquiry. Unlike natural scientists and many social scientists, criminologists tend to be scattered thinly, operating within departments and organisations which bear another title: law, or psychiatry, or sociology, or policy, or psychology, and so on. Few start their intellectual life seeing themselves as criminologists; many do not stay for ever within this specialty; some never accept the label of criminologist. They are attracted in by many motives, but prime among them seems to be the challenge of crime or offending to the ways of operating of their first discipline. People become tantalised or perplexed by deviance, by crime, by the difficulty of dealing with crime, by the challenge of the power wielded by the state in proscribing and controlling it. In different countries, the dominant routes into criminology differ and so the techniques and skills that are imported also differ.

The skills imported from law, or from sociology, form one aspect of the culture of criminological enquiry in a country. But there are other aspects which are sometimes less obvious, but none the less form the mind-set influencing which questions are seen as most relevant, and which solutions the most obvious. The social and legal culture of a country is also crucial. We grow up with assumptions about the place of law, the proper structure of a criminal justice system, the major dangers that come with power, the likely routes for expression of deviance. We grow up with particular ideas about the role and the nature of the state which are fundamental to the expression of criminal justice and the nature of crime (Dyson 1980). These ideas and assumptions are the bedrock of professional 'understandings' between professionals concerned with crime.

Criminology has never been entirely constrained by national boundaries, or practised within a country entirely by its own nationals – so there has always been questioning, and, as the pace of professional movement between European countries quickens after 1992, there will be more questioning. But the cultural traditions remain strong, as can be seen in any European seminar or committee discussing criminal matters. They lead to people using the same words, but hearing them with different conceptual baggage attached. In a European forum, there has to be a struggle to explain this baggage before there can be meaningful communication. This can be achieved and, increasingly, it is achieved. As the literature and practices of different countries become more accessible, the process will become easier.

Some may say that this is over-pessimistic. It is certainly true that ideas born in one country have swept through others, particularly at the beginning of criminological enquiry, when the views of Ferri, Durkheim, Garofalo, Bonger, Mannheim, Radzinowicz and others were seized upon in many countries, despite the fact that face-to-face meetings and communication were far more difficult than today. Have we developed, paradoxically, a situation where, despite our plethora of conferences and paper, our mental barriers have become stronger, our inner prejudices more exclusionary? Perhaps the more recent focus on enquiry at a local and micro-level, on quantitative empirical study, on policy which must necessarily be tied into cultural specifics, has enclosed criminologists in mental envelopes.

The definite wish for a more European understanding that has come about in the last few years may be a reaction to all this. We know there is interesting activity going on in other countries. We want to know about it, to try to understand. Some fear this process – that it will lead to a homogenisation of thought, driven by the more powerful interests. Some say that a particular brand of thought which they themselves dislike will be exported to other places, there to multiply, grow and strangle native-born enquiry, like some variety of triffid. They point to the powerful influence of American criminology (though the particular variety dominant at any time has never managed to stifle the heterogeneity of Europe). They fear that, say, administrative criminology, policy-linked and directed towards influencing the behaviour of those who offend, may become the uniform model for criminology and criminal justice policy. Such a uniformity would indeed induce stasis and limit the possibility for change and development.

This debate, however, seems to be a more modern, European, version of the perennial one – What is criminology? Either we welcome its plurality and accept its bittiness and lack of cohesion. Or we long for a strong guiding set of principles, a strong school of thought, though this will promote difficulty in producing change and produce a tendency towards painful revolution, rather than gradual movement, when change becomes necessary.

We have seen that the particular culture of a country has shaped its criminologists and its criminologies. Particular countries are, as a result, now famed for particular methodological strengths. Where there is a group of those interested in criminology who have been trained in one discipline, and where national conditions allow relevant access to criminal justice or social institutions, then younger scholars can learn within a strong tradition. A particular form of study becomes the expected form and there is a body of people able to criticise new work and drive forward developments. Empirical work, particularly, requires access and funding, if it is not to be constrained to solitary work by lone individuals.

Where there is a tradition of a particular kind of work, then links will be forged with the relevant interested policy-makers and funders and that tradition will be strengthened. But where there are such close links, change in the subject will be promoted not only within the discourse of academics, but also by the needs of policy. Change in schools of thought may become faster to accommodate the typically much shorter time-scales of administrators and politicians.

TRADITIONS AND STRENGTHS

These cultural traditions have shaped different strengths in different countries and fora. The international institutes, for example, such as the Max-Planck-Institute or HEUNI (the relevant United Nations-affiliated Institute for Information exchange in Europe) have major strengths in the comparative analysis of law and of criminal justice practice (see e.g. Joutsen 1987; Heine and Meinberg 1989). The Council of Europe is able to draw upon scholars from different countries and persuade governments to fill in questionnaires on the topics chosen for its conferences and its committees. The various Recommendations and Conventions therefore usually contain, in their explanatory reports, a résumé of comparative law and criminal justice system practice for those countries (see e.g. Council of Europe 1985, 1987). Without the access to materials provided by a structure which brings together experts from different countries conversant with the relevant literature, comparative research is made very difficult.

In the Federal Republic of Germany, a number of factors have promoted a strong tradition of legal scholarship, which has been able to be turned into studies exploring the criminal process and alternatives to the current criminal justice system and penal law, using both empirical methods and theoretical and philosophical exploration. The federal system, with the Länder having considerable jurisdiction in the criminal and penal law fields, has enabled experimentation in criminal process and police and court practices. The strength of law faculties and the interchange of both people and ideas between policy-makers and the academic sector has also promoted discussion of current issues. The result recently has been almost an explosion of interest in criminological and criminal justice topics. The topics are numerous, but include exploring the effects of the legal process on its participants, for example victims (e.g. Sessar 1982), explorations of alternative models for the courts (e.g. Jung 1989), projects on the prison population and on regimes (Graham 1988) and an interest in crime prevention, much of it locally focused at the city level (Jager 1989).

Indeed, the criminal justice system has been a focus in many countries. Almost all have some researchers working on topics such as the response by the police to calls from the public (e.g. Enhus and Hendrieckx 1988); or the reactions of victims (e.g. Killias 1989 in Switzerland; Newburn 1988 in England); or the functions and problematics of policing (e.g. Fijnaut and Hermans 1987). Indeed, the emerging interest in Eastern Europe in criminological matters is targeted on criminal justice (see Bienkowska, Chapter 4 in this volume), as well as juvenile delinquency and crime prevention (Graham 1990a).

In Eastern Europe, there is now a growing interest in criminological research. As we noted above, the institutions and culture of criminal justice and social control are related to the model of the state adopted in particular countries. In Eastern Europe, the extent of ownership of problems by the state extends to ownership of the problem of crime and delinquency. The state hence has responsibility for dealing with crime – and so everyone has responsibility for it, rather than such responsibility being confined to certain sectors or occupational groups. Everyone – every individual – equally has responsibility for areas of social control, and so one finds a blurring of tasks and responsibilities between the more obvious agencies of formal social control, such as the police and courts, and other groupings based on the work-place and neighbourhood. In the USSR, for example, considerable use is made of lay tribunals and voluntary police (Graham 1989) and crime prevention includes a system of 'neighbourhood watch' in flats entirely organised by flat-dwellers. Equally, as Los (1989) has shown, the state economy and the 'black economy' are comprehensively inter-linked. This brings into play different ideas of the place of law and the subject-matter of criminology: economic models, regulatory justice, the idea of treating offenders as showing symptoms of something wrong with the communal situation, leading to courts acting on the agencies shaping the situation of the individual rather than just punishing the individual.

In western Europe, there has been a much greater focus on

formal agencies of social control – on the state institutions of police, courts, prisons. But there has still been a struggling, small tradition of work on the informal, on small areas, on the ways communities live and cope with crime. This has often existed on the margins of anthropology, sociology and social geography – but it has a long history, particularly in England (see Downes 1989). It is necessarily area-bound and dependent upon researchers living and working in those areas for sufficient lengths of time. Often, therefore, the studies produced have had to stand alone; a snapshot of social control and crime in one place at one time (see e.g. Sprott *et al.* 1954; Shapland and Vagg 1988). Theoretical development has correspondingly proceeded in fits and starts. Insights have not always been followed up, usually not because of deliberate choice, but because such study is necessarily field-based and therefore dependent upon the dedication and inclinations of individuals – often research students. Occasionally, however, it has been possible to follow the changes wrought in one area for much longer and pull out the much richer and more explanatory dynamic processes involved in changes in patterns of behaviour and in the pressures exerted by reputations, local bureaucratic practices and social pressures. A notable example is the study of crime and housing in Sheffield (see Bottoms *et al.* 1987; Bottoms and Wiles 1988).

In France, the history of criminological enquiry has been one of periods of considerable interest, followed by more fallow patches, where academic interest has switched back to more mainstream concerns within sociology, law and history. Currently, as in all countries in Europe, there is a major boom – but the diverse activity being undertaken has retained its connections with its parent discipline. There is less danger here of an atheoretical empiricism or fieldwork being driven solely by short-term policy goals. The dominant feature is links with ideas of the history of the social and political development of the mainstream culture. Links do not need to be forged with political scientists or historians; criminological work is steeped in those traditions. None the less, the growing plurality of subject areas and methods will throw in alien influences and it is currently difficult to see the resulting theoretical trends. The most recent moves have been to tie up ideas about the political/social/historical nexus with empirical work using surveys, observation, analysis of statistical data, and in-depth interviewing, on very different areas of the criminal justice system: victim experiences (e.g. Zauberman 1985); the courts (Zauberman 1989); the state police (Monjardet 1988).

In Britain, there has also been a fascination with the processes and systems of criminal justice – but often at the level of the agency, rather than in relation to wider cultural and political movements. The police, for example, tend to be studied in and of themselves, rather like peering into an ant colony isolated by glass and placed in a museum (see Shapland and Hobbs 1989). The placing and relationship of the various 'exhibits' are rarely studied, though more statistically and model-oriented work from the Home Office and others has started to lay bare the interrelationships (see Moxon 1985).

None the less, this tradition of detailed examination of institutions has left a rich collection of studies of discretion, decision-making, institutional pressures, accountability, the relationship of policy and practice (Rock 1988a). It has also informed theoretical developments, most of which have been based firmly in sociological models and traditions. Naturally the focus of these has changed as wider political and social movements have changed (though these links have rarely been made explicit). The concern has moved from ideas of treatment, based on the individual, through ideas about social control and its use by the state and dominant classes (see Taylor *et al.* 1973) to a more heterogeneous set of concepts: the interaction of the state's setting apart of criminals and their own views of themselves; accountability of institutions to the political process (see Morgan 1987) and to individual consumers (e.g. Shapland *et al.* 1985); the internal dynamics of the professions; attempts to affect criminal behaviour through changing the environment, especially in England (see Hope and Shaw 1988b); and even attempts to understand the policy-making process itself (see Rock 1988b). Scotland and Northern Ireland have similarly heterogeneous experiences, but there the focuses, given the more limited quantity of work, have been more discrete.

The volume of work in Britain, particularly on the empirical side, has always been high. Criminology has embraced researchers and theorists from many disciplines and such an inter-disciplinary exchange of views is now institutionalised in many of the outlets and structures – the Cambridge Institute of Criminology, the British Society of Criminology, the British Journal of Criminology and many others, all of which contain and wish to continue to contain inputs from many different kinds of research. In such a pluralist and pragmatic culture, tensions are normal, though their focus varies over time. Sometimes there have been great theoretical debates within criminology itself. At others there has been difficulty between researcher and agencies over access, or over control of the findings of the research and their dissemination. At others, notably the present time, there are difficulties of understanding between academic sector and government about the place of each other and each other's proper role. Britain has always been a recipient of ideas from North America and that does not look like changing. It is now beginning to be influenced to a much greater degree by other European criminologies – and the future looks more heterogeneous, and exciting.

The Netherlands have seen a similar pluralism of criminological method and of culture, but the strands have been slightly different and the theoretical and empirical interaction between different researchers perhaps less total. Here it has been possible until recently to keep together for considerable periods of time clearly differentiated groups of thinkers and researchers in particular institutions and university departments. Schools of thought have been able to develop in particular places, rather than being washed by the tide of time over more scattered individual researchers. One tradition has been the development of empirical research on victimisation, attitudes about crime, crime prevention projects, the use of law, and criminal justice professionals' practices – using large samples, strict experimental action research evaluation designs, and relatively sophisticated statistical methods. Psychology, particularly social psychological techniques and theories drawn from North America, has been a major influence, not only in university departments (see e.g. Winkel 1987), but also in the Ministry of Justice research unit. That unit is large and has produced an impressive volume of work (see Junger-Tas and Block 1988; van Dijk 1988a). It has formed a linchpin of funding and of inspiring work, both complementary work and work deliberately designed to provide a very different and alternative focus. Some of the latter has included the abolitionist school and the focus on informal dispute resolution.

Standing outside Scandinavia, it is tempting to see Scandinavian criminology as an entity, especially since there is continuous dialogue between the countries, institutionalised in councils and written output. But that would be a major mistake. There has always been a heterogeneity of work and different traditions there. Some has clear legal roots, developing out of a tradition of analysis of the codified penal law. Other work has concentrated upon empirical study of particular phenomena, such as the Swedish National Crime Prevention Council. There has also been a willingness to invest many years of effort in longitudinal studies on offending and changes by age and with social residence variables – both in locality studies and in studies of individuals (for example, the studies of twins Christiansen [1974; 1977]). In smaller countries, criminology by definition has to be carried on by individuals, interacting as much with scholars in similar fields outside the country as within it. In the Scandinavian countries, this distancing effect has been effectively counteracted by the formation of institutes and structures to promote particular foci of work. It is a model which could be adopted with advantage in the wider and opening arena of Europe.

Though there is some concentration on individual offenders in some countries, notably the Netherlands, the prime focus in Europe is on the social: the collectivity, the agency, the state. In Italy, however, there is a strong and enduring tradition of focus upon the individual, arising out of a fascination with the deviant and the disturbed. Strong bonds exist between law and psychiatry, going back to the work of Lombroso. Much work has followed a tradition of psychiatric and psychological enquiry into the dilemmas intrinsic to the interaction of medicine and the law – competing ideas of the dangerous, incapacitation versus treatment, the consequences for individuals. Some of it has adopted the paradigms of mainstream psychiatry and law; some rebelled against these, leading to the abolition of mental institutions and the anti-psychiatry movement (see Reali and Shapland 1986). Equally in reaction, there has been a separate tradition of relatively abstract sociological enquiry at the level of discourse about the nature of state in society. In Italy and in a few other places, the tradition of the individual and the idea that there are individual differences has been kept alive. It may be an idea that may sweep back over Europe soon.

BACK TO THE FUTURE

In this brief and inevitably perfunctory review of criminology in Europe, it has been possible and even necessary to write in terms of countries. The barriers of borders are still strong; the discourses turning inwards to national capitals rather than reaching out to an international network. The barriers of language are still there. Academic prestige and academic training are to be found in national universities and institutions. More constraining are the hidden barriers: those of culture, legal tradition, methodological correctness, implicit notions of state, justice, structures, community and social order.

But there are powerful forces pushing against all those barriers. As Heidensohn writes in Chapter 1, there is an eagerness amongst policy-makers, amongst empirical paymasters, amongst intellectual enquirers, to surmount the barriers and gain an understanding of what is on the other side. So shall we move towards a uniform and homogeneous European criminology? In some areas, probably yes. The similarities between the needs of consumers of criminal justice institutions in different legal systems, and the similar goals of policy-makers, are likely to make criminal justice research and criminal justice experiments more rather than less uniform. The year 1992 will increase contact as professionals move more freely around. We may start believing that all should speak more than one language as a matter of course. It is to be hoped, however, the pressures towards progress will recognise the benefits of difference for experiment and for analysis. We may see both a localisation and a wider uniformity in criminal justice.

In other areas of enquiry, I feel it is highly unlikely that criminology will become uniform. Perhaps more prone to radical change, perhaps less insular, as we may move back to a time when schools of thought can spread more easily than now. But it will never become homogeneous: its very nature as a between subject – between law, sociology, psychology, psychiatry, geography, politics and many others – will ensure that.

© 1991 Joanna Shapland

Part two

Patterns and Trends

Chapter three

More than a matter of security

Trends in crime prevention in Europe

Jan van Dijk

INTRODUCTION

Governments across Europe increasingly collaborate with each other in economic, financial and social policies. In the area of crime policies, however, each of the European countries is still very much doing its own thing without giving much attention to developments elsewhere. In some respects crime policies of the main European countries are quite different from one another. In spite of the variety in organisational structures and policies, some common trends can still be discerned. In most countries, for instance, the interest in preventive policies has grown since the mid-1980s.

In this chapter I shall first present some data about the development, size and nature of the crime problem in European countries. I shall look at trends in rates of registered or officially recorded crime and at the results of an international victimisation survey. Next I shall compare national expenditures on policing and prisons with those on crime prevention (private security, household security measures and governmental crime prevention programmes). In a final section an assessment will be made of the state-of-the-art of crime prevention in Europe so far and of the prospects for new policies in the 1990s.

CRIME AND VICTIMISATION RATES

In order to put national crime prevention policies in a proper perspective, it is essential to look at national crime figures first. Many inhabitants of European countries tend to see rising crime rates as a sort of national curse. This opinion is not borne out by the facts, as can readily be seen from a survey of the statistics on recorded crime of five European countries since 1950 (see Figure 3.1).

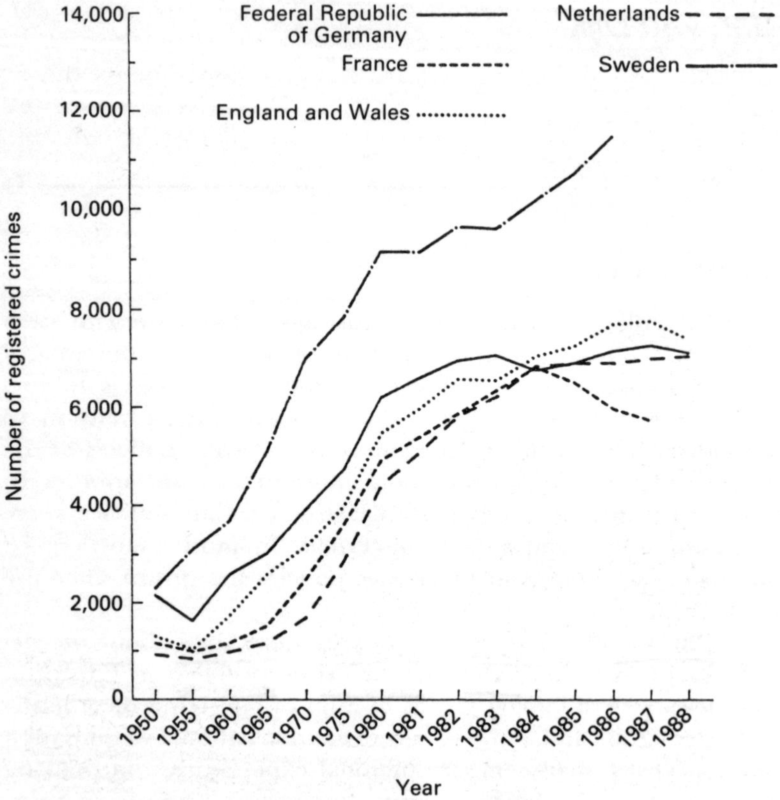

Sources: Official police statistics:
Rechtsbescherming en veiligheid CBS;
Criminal Statistics England and Wales;
Polizeiliche Kriminalstatistik;
Beveilgings jaarboek 1984 bldz 15 en 1989 bldz 12, en Annual;
Yearbook of Nordic Statistics 1986, table 229.

Figure 3.1 Registered crime in five European countries per 100,000 inhabitants

Most European nations have experienced sharp rises in registered crime over the past three decades. Between 1985 and 1986 registered crime in France, England and Wales, the Federal Republic of Germany (FRG) and the Netherlands seems to have reached a ceiling around the rate of 7,000 registered crimes per 100,000 inhabitants.

A closer analysis of the police figures shows that property crimes are particularly high in Sweden and the Netherlands. Crimes of violence, though, are recorded much more often by the police in Sweden, the FRG and England and Wales (see Figure 3.2).

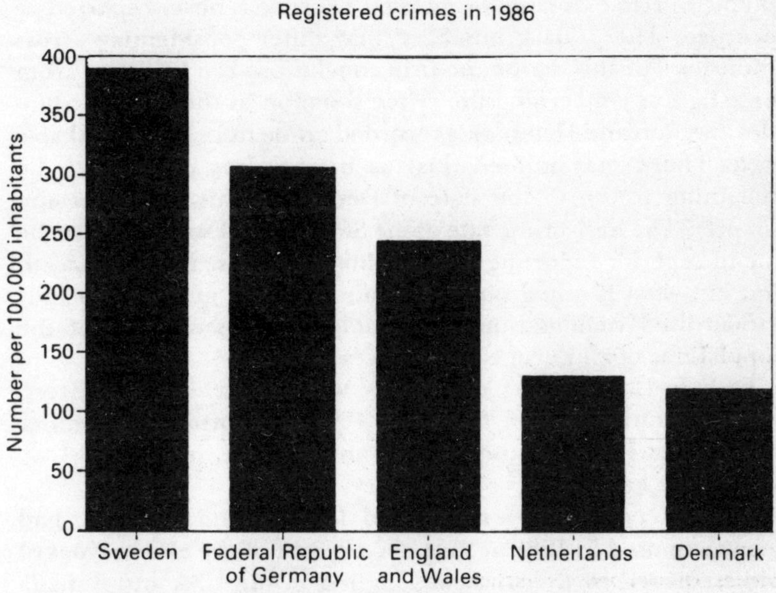

Sources: Official police statistics:
Rechtsbescherming en veiligheid CBS;
Criminal Statistics England and Wales;
Polizeiliche Kriminalstatistik;
Yearbook of Nordic Statistics 1986, table 229

Figure 3.2 Violence against the person

Compared with the homicide rate of 10 per 100,000 inhabitants in the USA, the number of homicides in western European countries is still very low (between 0.5 and 1.5 per 100,000 according to the World Health Organization, 1984).

In England and Wales and the Netherlands the rates for crimes of violence have continued to rise in the past three years. The rate for crimes of violence went from 133 to 148 in 1988 in the Netherlands and from 282 to 315 in England and Wales. This recent trend may foreshadow a gradual change in the crime pattern in Europe. A somewhat larger proportion of recorded registered crime in Europe may consist of violent crime in the 1990s.

It goes without saying that police statistics do not reflect the true volume of crime. A large proportion of crime is never reported or recorded. These 'dark numbers' may differ considerably across countries. For this reason, no firm conclusions can be drawn from these figures concerning the crime situation in the various countries. Sweden and Denmark's recorded crime rates are remarkably high. There may indeed, just as in the days of Hamlet, be something rotten in the state of Denmark. This is not certain, however. The high crime rate of the Swedes and Danes may also be due to superior reporting or recording practices. The only way to find out what is going on in Scandinavia is by mounting a fully standardised victimisation survey amongst cross-sections of the populations of all European countries.

Early in 1989 a survey of this type was conducted in seventeen different countries (van Dijk *et al.* 1990). Unfortunately neither Sweden nor Denmark took part in this venture. In Table 3.1 we present the key findings of the survey.

The percentage of persons aged 16 years and over who had been victimised in 1988 at least once by one of the eleven types of crime covered by the study was highest in the USA and Canada (approx. 30 per cent).

Countries with overall victimisation rates of about 25 per cent were Australia, the Netherlands, Spain and the FRG. A victimisation rate of about 20 per cent was found in Scotland, England and Wales, France and Belgium. Rates in the neighbourhood of 15 per cent were found amongst the public of Northern Ireland, Switzerland, Norway and Finland.

Countries with the lowest rates are characterised by a relatively low level of urbanisation, that is many of their inhabitants live in small villages and few in cities with 100,000 inhabitants or more.

Crimes of violence appeared to be the highest in Australia and the USA. Moderately high victimisation rates for violence were found in Finland, the Netherlands, the FRG, Canada and Scotland. In England and Wales the rates were significantly lower than elsewhere.

The ranking of countries on the basis of victimisation rates is not vastly different from the picture shown by police figures. The overall victimisation rates in England and Wales are somewhat lower than was to be expected on the basis of Interpol statistics. This is not accounted for by a significantly higher percentage of crimes reported to the police in the UK. The relatively high police figures could reflect high victimisation rates among shops, schools and other institutions. Recording practices of the police could be different in the UK as well.

This overview of official crime rates and victimisation rates leads to the following tentative conclusions. Crime has gone up from 1955 onwards across western Europe. In Sweden the upward trend started immediately after the war. At the end of the 1980s crimes like theft, burglary, simple assault and indecent assault place a heavy burden on the inhabitants of the larger European cities in particular. On average however, the crime problem is still less serious than in the USA.

EXPENDITURES ON CRIME PREVENTION AND CONTROL

Since the level of crime is fairly similar across the main European countries, one might expect expenditures on crime policies to be rather similar as well. In Table 3.2 some key figures on these expenditures are presented. We have collected data from various sources on the expenditures on both the criminal justice system (police and prisons) and the prevention of crime.

The Federal Republic of Germany employs the highest number of police officers per capita. Fewer police officers are available in the Netherlands and Sweden. Expenditures on the prison system are the highest in Sweden and England and Wales. High expenditures in Sweden are caused by high costs per prisoner (147 prison guards per 100 prisoners, compared with 53 in England and Wales, 42 in the FRG, 41 in France and 96 in the Netherlands). The imprisonment rates in England and Wales are presently the highest in western Europe – 95 per 100,000 of the population (in Australia the rate is 105). This explains the high expenditures on

Table 3.1 Victimisation rates for fourteen countries and for Europe, the total of the fourteen countries, and rates for Warsaw and Surabaja [a]

	Car theft		*Theft from car*		*Car vandalism*		*Motor theft*		*Bike theft*		*Burglary*		*Attempt burglary*		*Violent theft*		*Other theft*		*Sexual offence* [b]		*Attack or threat*		*All crimes* [c]
	1988	*5 yrs*	*1988*	*5 yrs*	*1988*	*5 yrs*	*1988*	*5 yrs*	*1988*	*5 yrs*	*1988*	*5 yrs*	*1988*	*5 yrs*	*1988*	*5 yrs*	*1988*	*5 yrs*	*1988*	*5 yrs*	*1988*	*5 yrs*	*1988*
Total	1,2	4,2	5,3	14,8	6,7	16,9	0,4	1,2	2,6	9,6	2,1	7,8	2,0	6,6	0,9	3,1	4,0	11,9	2,5	6,3	2,9	7,8	21,1
Europe	1,3	4,6	5,8	16,6	7,0	18,6	0,4	1,5	2,2	8,5	1,8	7,3	1,9	6,6	1,0	3,6	3,9	12,0	1,9	5,6	2,5	7,4	20,9
England and Wales	1,8	6,6	5,6	13,4	6,8	17,3	0,0	0,4	1,0	3,9	2,1	9,4	1,7	6,0	0,7	1,9	3,1	8,3	1,2	3,4	1,9	5,3	19,4
Scotland	0,8	5,3	5,3	12,9	6,5	14,9	0,3	0,4	1,0	3,1	2,0	9,0	2,1	5,8	0,5	1,8	2,6	6,7	1,2	2,9	1,8	5,3	18,6
N.Ireland	1,6	5,2	4,0	8,5	4,5	10,3	0,2	0,4	1,6	4,0	1,1	4,7	0,9	2,9	0,5	1,5	2,2	6,1	1,8	3,3	1,8	4,3	15,0
Netherlands	0,3	1,8	5,3	15,2	8,2	21,6	0,4	1,3	7,6	24,8	2,4	8,9	2,6	9,3	0,9	2,0	4,5	14,3	2,6	6,4	3,4	9,3	26,8
FRG	0,4	1,9	4,7	14,8	8,7	22,1	0,2	0,9	3,3	12,4	1,3	4,7	1,8	5,6	0,8	3,0	3,9	13,3	2,8	7,9	3,1	9,3	21,9
Switzerland	0,0	0,9	1,9	8,4	4,1	13,4	1,2	4,1	3,2	12,8	1,0	4,0	0,2	2,1	0,5	2,2	4,5	15,9	1,6	5,5	1,2	3,9	15,6

Belgium	0,8	4,0	2,7	8,7	6,6	17,9	0,3	1,4	2,7	9,8	2,3	7,7	2,3	8,2	1,0	4,0	4,0	14,9	1,3	4,9	2,0	6,4	17,7
France	2,3	7,3	6,0	21,0	6,5	19,6	0,6	2,9	1,4	6,6	2,4	10,4	2,3	8,9	0,4	2,9	3,6	12,8	1,2	4,3	2,0	7,1	19,4
Spain	1,3	5,0	9,9	24,6	6,3	16,0	0,8	2,3	1,0	3,3	1,7	5,6	1,9	6,9	2,8	9,1	5,0	13,4	2,4	6,8	3,0	7,5	24,6
Norway	1,1	2,7	2,8	9,0	4,6	11,2	0,3	0,6	2,8	12,5	0,8	3,2	0,4	2,3	0,5	1,5	3,2	8,3	2,1	4,7	3,0	8,2	16,5
Finland	0,4	1,7	2,7	8,2	4,0	10,5	0,0	0,2	3,1	14,1	0,6	2,0	0,4	2,2	0,8	2,7	4,3	10,3	0,6	4,3	2,9	9,7	15,9
USA	2,1	6,3	9,3	26,7	8,9	21,7	0,2	0,5	3,1	9,4	3,8	13,7	5,4	13,5	1,9	5,5	4,5	14,2	4,5	10,4	5,4	12,7	28,8
Canada	0,8	2,8	7,2	18,5	9,8	18,8	0,3	0,6	3,4	12,4	3,0	10,2	2,7	7,9	1,1	2,6	5,4	13,2	4,0	10,0	4,0	8,8	28,1
Australia	2,3	8,0	6,9	17,2	8,7	20,8	0,2	0,5	1,9	5,8	4,4	16,6	3,8	11,6	0,9	2,3	5,0	14,6	7,3	13,5	5,2	11,6	27,8
Warsaw	2,2	4,6	10,2	19,8	7,6	16,0	0,0	0,0	1,0	4,6	2,6	9,0	2,8	10,8	1,2	4,6	13,4	27,0	3,6	7,2	3,0	7,4	
Surabaja	0,2	0,3	4,7	11,0	2,7	5,7	0,8	2,8	2,7	11,0	3,8	11,5	1,7	5,2	0,5	2,8	5,2	16,0	6,3	14,3	0,8	4,2	

Notes: a The survey was held during the early months of 1989 and the respondents were asked if they had been the victim of a crime during the past 5 years; and if so they were asked whether the incident happened in 1989 or 1988 or before 1988.

b The question about sexual offences was put to women only.

c In 'All crimes 1988' the percentage of respondents who have been the victim of one or more crimes in 1988 is given.

Source: Van Dijk *et al.* 1990.

prisons in the UK. In the FRG rates of imprisonment have gone down considerably during the past five years; the rate is now around 80, just as in France. In Sweden the rate is 49, and in the Netherlands, 36.

Table 3.2 Indicators of annual expenditure on crime policies in five European countries in the mid-1980s, per 100,000 inhabitants in million $

	Police officers	*Private security officers*	*Prisons*	*Household security measures expenditures*	*Expenditure on crime prevention*	*Total*
FRG	12.4	8.0	1.5	0.42		22.3
France	10.4	5.2	0.8	0.42	0.01	16.8
England and Wales	10.0	8.4	2.2	0.34	0.02	21.0
Netherlands	9.6	3.0	1.0	0.28	0.04	13.9
Sweden	7.2	10.0	2.7	0.42	0.02	20.3

Note: The annual costs per police officer and private security officer are estimated at $40,000 for all countries.

Sources: HEUNI 1985; Council of Europe 1988a; Frost and Sullivan Ltd 1988; Ministry of Justice 1984; van Dijk 1988b; Home Office 1988a.

Private security is much more prominent in Sweden, the FRG and England and Wales than in France and the Netherlands. The rates of household security sales are less divergent, but somewhat lower in England and again in the Netherlands. Government expenditures on crime prevention are modest in comparison to those on prisons and police forces across Europe. The expenditures on crime prevention are extremely low in the FRG, since federal programmes do not exist and only some of the states have developed concrete policies. The expenditures in the UK are largely part of other government programmes such as employment schemes. Expenditures on Home Office crime prevention projects are of marginal importance (approx. $0.02 million per 100,000 inhabitants, mainly spent on mass media campaigns). By comparison the annual expenditure of around $0.04 million in the Netherlands seems rather high. The Dutch expenditures have been politically justified with reference to the even higher expenditures which would be required for criminal justice if prevention were not promoted adequately.

It is clear from the data in Table 3.1 that the Federal Republic of Germany spends somewhat more than other countries on crime prevention and control and the Netherlands and Sweden substantially less. To our knowledge, expenditures on the judiciary exhibit the same pattern, with particularly high costs in the FRG. Somewhat surprisingly, the level of expenditures on crime policies shows more variation across the main European countries than the volume of recorded crimes. There is no clear relationship of any kind between the level of expenditures on criminal justice and the level of recorded crime. Expenditures in England and Wales, for instance, are rather high, but victimisation rates are relatively low. The FRG has high crime and victimisation rates as well as high expenditures. The Netherlands combines high victimisation rates with substantially lower expenditures than elsewhere in Europe.

CRIME PREVENTION AND THE CAUSES OF CRIME

The recent history of crime prevention policies has not been quite the same in the various western countries but some general patterns can still be discerned. In the 1960s crime prevention was often equated with programmes of social reform (Jeffery 1977). It was advocated as an alternative to the punitive policies of the criminal justice authorities. The dominant notion was that crime could be cured by better housing, schooling, welfare and employment policies.

The trends in recorded crime in western Europe seem to indicate a real increase in the number of crimes committed since 1955. This upward trend runs parallel to a gradual rise in affluence, social security, quality of housing, level of education and health services across western Europe. This obvious positive correlation between levels of crime and levels of prosperity cannot be reconciled easily with the conventional criminological wisdom that poverty breeds crime. On the contrary, the western European experience suggests that crime rates go up jointly with the Gross National Product (GNP).

The ranking of European nations in terms of victimisation rates or official crime rates does not lend support to the 'poverty breeds crime' thesis either. The most affluent societies have not been blessed with low levels of crime. Among countries with the highest GNP per capita are several countries with high crime or victimisation rates, notably the USA, Canada, the FRG and Sweden. Countries with high GNPs but low crime/victimisation rates are Switzerland and Finland. Spain is a clear example of a country with a low GNP and a high victimisation rate. There seems to be a weak *positive* correlation between GNP and crime levels.

It is beyond the scope of this chapter to explain the social mechanisms behind this correlation. Three factors seem to be important. First, in a more affluent and democratic society, those who are less well off may resent the obvious inequality more vehemently. Second, affluence and social security make young people less dependent upon their families and state institutions; this may lessen social control. Third, affluence simply creates greater opportunities for property crimes. Whatever may be the determining factors, surely the experience of western Europe since the 1950s undermines the belief that crime will automatically dwindle if more affluent and equal societies are established. If social justice is seen as the cure to crime, this seems to be a long-term option only.

In the 1970s the concept of crime prevention through social reform gradually lost its credibility. Since the preventive concept had failed, expenditures on criminal justice system were expanded in many countries (Young 1988).

At the same time, several governments established committees of experts to reassess their policies of crime prevention and control. Examples of such committees are the Peyrefitte Committee of 1977 and the Bonnemaison Committee of 1982 in France and the Roethof Committee of 1983 in the Netherlands. Although each of these committees worked in splendid isolation, their recommendations were nevertheless very much alike. Each recommended a strengthening of the national government's commitment to crime prevention, inter-agency co-operation at the local level and a greater involvement of private citizens and businesses. This involvement was to go beyond the use of technical devices.

As a follow-up to these recommendations, Sweden, Denmark, France and, more recently, Belgium, have set up national crime prevention councils with representatives from various ministries.

In both the UK and the Netherlands inter-departmental groups were set up to steer the new crime prevention policies. The Federal Republic of Germany seems to be the exception to the rule that new national bodies for the promotion of crime prevention policies were set up between 1975 and 1985.

On the advice of these various committees new, more specific kinds of crime prevention policies evolved. Crime prevention was no longer viewed as just one of the positive side-effects of the Welfare State but acquired a separate identity. Under the banner of crime prevention, activities became fashionable which did not aim at (pre)delinquents but at those at risk of being *victimised* by crime. Crime prevention became victim-oriented.

The new buzz words were target hardening, crime prevention through environmental design, defensible space, situational crime prevention and opportunity reduction (Newman 1972; Mayhew *et al.* 1976; Brantingham and Brantingham 1981; Kube 1986). It was subsequently understood that, in order to be effective, such measures need to be combined with organised surveillance (van Dijk and Junger-Tas 1988; Rosenbaum 1988). A second wave of crime prevention initiatives in the 1980s aimed to strengthen informal social control by means of neighbourhood watch, private security, caretakers, etc. (Hope and Shaw 1988a).

The common element of victim-oriented crime prevention is that potential victims are exhorted to take measures to protect themselves against criminal risks. Crime policy is no longer the exclusive responsibility of the state. Several typologies of such protective, defensive or community crime prevention measures are proposed in the literature. A distinction is often made between technical and social measures (techno-prevention and socio-prevention). Another important distinction is between measures taken by individuals and those taken by social groups.

On the basis of these two criteria a typology can be constructed as presented in Table 3.3.

PROSPECTS AND LIMITATIONS OF VICTIM-ORIENTED CRIME PREVENTION PROSPECTS

Crime prevention in western Europe has been dominated since the 1970s by the concept of protection against criminal threats, as it has been in North America. While expenditures on crime prevention by both the private and public sector have gone up in the

1980s, there is still ample scope for further growth. Insurance companies seem ready to promote secondary crime prevention more actively. Market research predicts a continuous annual growth of 10 per cent in household security equipment. Similar growth rates are expected by private security firms. Plant managers are becoming increasingly aware of the economic importance of crime prevention as a part of a wider risk control policy, also covering the protection of computerised data (van Soomeren 1989). Local governments have likewise been sensitised to the importance of crime prevention as part of their efforts to improve the quality of life in urban areas. The number of neighbourhood schemes is rapidly expanding in the UK. In continental Europe surveillance is strengthened by the employment of more caretakers, bus conductors, city wardens, etc.

Victim-oriented crime prevention seems not yet to have reached its full practical potential. Many governments are still hesitant to invest serious money in it. Field and Hope (1989) have persuasively argued on economic grounds for government subsidies in the market for primary crime prevention. Other important priorities for government are research and development, the development of European standards and better regulation of the activities of private security firms.

Table 3.3 Typology of victim-oriented crime prevention strategies

	Individuals	*Social institutions*
Technical	locks and bolts burglar alarms	CCTV urban design
Social	neighbourhood watch	private security professional surveillance

EFFECTIVENESS OF PROTECTIVE MEASURES

Evaluation research on target hardening and other forms of victim-oriented prevention has so far yielded ambiguous results (Mayhew 1984; Rosenbaum 1988; E.H. Johnson 1987; Lab 1988). Neighbourhood watch programmes have been found to reduce burglary in the Netherlands but less so in England and Wales

(Savormin Lohman and van Dijk 1988; Bennett 1988). The ability to reduce specific types of criminal activities in specific situations if sufficient measures are taken, has been demonstrated clearly (van Andel 1989; Colder 1988). The value of such effects is often limited, however, by a displacement of the avoided crimes to other locations or by the substitution of new types of crimes. Displacement or substitution effects are no ground for a general debunking of victim-oriented prevention. It should be acknowledged that successful offender-oriented prevention may have more lasting benefits for the community at large.

NEGATIVE SIDE-EFFECTS

Fear reduction has been defined here as part of crime prevention. In practice, the relationship between crime and fear reduction is far from simple. Some measures or policies may serve both goals. Some may serve one of them exclusively. Another possibility is that certain policies have positive results in one area but compound problems in others.

Several victim-oriented policies have been found to reduce fear, without having a measurable impact upon crime levels (Fowler *et al.* 1979). Security surveys, crime prevention information campaigns, the redesigning of neighbourhoods and community projects have sometimes been found to lead to intensified fear (Winkel 1987; Rosenbaum 1988). Fear or anxiety should not always be interpreted as a social loss. In some situations it may even have important benefits. The fear-inducing side-effects of some victim-oriented prevention policies need always to be made part of their cost–benefits equation (Shapland and Vagg 1988). The gradual greying of the western European population in the next decades may make the side-effects of intensified fear more important, since elderly people are particularly sensitive to fear-invoking information.

SATURATION AND RESISTANCE

Although there is still scope for a further growth in the purchase of security measures in most western countries, it will become increasingly difficult to change the attitudes of those remaining parts of the population who have not yet been persuaded. To the extent that primary prevention has become more common, larger investments are required to bring about further growth. Mass media campaigns tend not to reach, or to affect, those least inclined to apply security measures (i.e. the ultimate target group of such campaigns). The younger population has a large share of individuals with an easy-going life-style. Risk-taking in all fields of life is part of their way of life. This part of the population seems to be highly resistant to the idea of protective measures. It has also become clear that neighbourhood watch programmes are much less popular with the urban population in continental Europe than in the UK, the USA and Canada. On the continent, neighbourhood watch is often disliked because of its association with the vigilantism of fascist organisations in the 1930s and 1940s.

A RENAISSANCE OF OFFENDER-ORIENTED CRIME PREVENTION

In recent years a series of criticisms has been levelled against victim-oriented crime prevention. Currie (1988) criticises the use of an often superficial concept of 'community' and the tendency to see criminals as dangerous outsiders who must be kept out of one's territory (the exclusionary vision). He also mentions the lack of awareness that offenders too are members of a community living in particular neighbourhoods.

Interestingly, similar ideas are floating around in the world of business security managers and consultants. Recent publications in the Netherlands and the UK about business security focus upon the internal sources of crime: theft and fraud by employees has become a new priority (Shapland and Wiles 1989). Crime prevention is consequently redefined as a part of broader social policies of companies covering the use of computers and safety measures and not as a specialised response to threats from the outside. In fact in some companies security, data security and safety are now presented as elements of a general quality control drive.

There are signs that crime prevention in at least some western societies will once again become oriented towards tackling the social problems which form the background of (serious) crime. The pendulum may soon start to swing back. In France, but also in Italy, crime prevention of the social reform type seems always to have retained its appeal (Waller 1989). In the UK and the Netherlands crime prevention is now relaunched as part of integrated urban renewal projects tackling unemployment, housing problems and crime in deteriorated city areas. In this new stage, some of the older preventive solutions may be given a better – and perhaps fairer – chance. More emphasis will probably be put on the importance of adequate socialisation processes and social control than in the 'anarchistic' 1960s (Currie 1988). Future buzz words may be normative training, self-discipline, data security, (electronic) surveillance and risk control. It is furthermore to be expected that the activities of private security companies and business security units will be viewed as part of a crime prevention policy (van Dijk 1989). At the Conference of Ministers of Justice of Council of Europe countries in The Hague in June 1989 several ministers expressed an interest in closer co-operation with the private security industry. European standards for private security services and practices will probably be developed in the years to come.

TO CONCLUDE

In many countries crime prevention policies in the period from 1975 to 1985 were largely of the victim-oriented type (locks and bolts, neighbourhood watch). At this stage, responsibility for crime prevention was largely put in the hands of the police as part of their public relations policies. Within an overall crime policy such activities were of marginal importance. A new situation arises if offender-oriented prevention policies become additional priorities. These new activities need to be co-ordinated with various activities of the criminal justice system (with the uniformed police, CID, prosecutions, after care, and so on). The concept of an integrated crime policy, the dream of nineteenth-century positivist criminology, becomes topical again. So too does the question of organisation 'ownership' or control over such a policy.

In my view, an integrated crime policy needs to be based upon a partnership between local government and the police. In many countries, the prosecution office will be the third party. At the national or state and federal level the Minister of Justice should be made responsible for co-ordination and support of local policies. The recent integration in France of the National Crime Prevention Council into a newly established National Council for Cities and Urban Social Development may signal a decreased interest of the French Government in crime prevention. Special subsidies for crime prevention projects are bound to be abolished (Faugeron 1989).

If the co-ordination of crime prevention policies does not lie with justice or police-based agencies, such policies run the risk of being abandoned as soon as the crime problem is off the political agenda. The mission of crime prevention agencies should be to remain active in periods with less acute crime problems, as do agencies monitoring traffic or industrial safety.

At all levels, concrete policies should start with an empirical assessment of the crime problem as an issue. Victimisation surveys and self-report delinquency studies are indispensable tools for such an assessment. Each of the identified crime problems will require a special mixture of various types of interventions. For instance, in the case of a high rate of armed robbery, the optimal mix might consist of

1 sophisticated protection of local banks, training of bank personnel concerning coping strategies;
2 victim support to actual victims;
3 criminal justice activities (special squad of the CID to investigate local gangs); and
4 offender-oriented prevention (after-care programmes for bank-robbers released from prison).

In the case of a high rate of vandalism against public property the optimal mix will of course be quite different. It may consist of special courses in primary schools (offender-oriented prevention), target hardening of public buildings at vulnerable spots (victim-oriented prevention) and community service orders for young vandals (criminal justice and offender-oriented prevention).

It is hoped that crime prevention in the 1990s is recognised as an indispensable component of a modern crime policy and that this leads to a better cost–benefit ratio in the fight against crime for all parties involved (offenders, victims and the government). Closer co-operation within Europe in this field may help to give crime prevention the academic and political impetus it needs to develop into an established part of government policies.[1] The time seems ripe for a European Crime Prevention Programme, to be sponsored by the European Social Fund, national governments and/or European companies.

© 1991 Jan van Dijk

Chapter four

Crime in eastern Europe[1]

Ewa Bienkowska

INTRODUCTION

The study of crime in a single country is fraught with difficulties, which are compounded when comparing crime in several countries. As we all know, crime statistics as provided by the police and the courts are a rather imperfect measure of actual crime levels. They tell us as much about reporting and recording procedures as they do about crime itself. Countries with different legal systems both define and record criminal acts in different ways. These differences are compounded further by an attempt to compare crime trends over time, as recording practices may change.

The study of crime in eastern Europe (Holyst 1979: 97ff) is subject to special difficulties. Access to statistics varies considerably within eastern Europe, both for the general public and for professionals and academics. We can identify four different scenarios.

1 Data are available neither to the public, nor to people who deal with crime problems professionally, e.g. Romania.
2 Limited access to data is available for research purposes, but requires special permission; however, such data cannot be cited or published, even for scientific purposes, e.g. the USSR.
3 Some rather superficial data are available for anyone interested in official and widely available statistical periodicals, e.g. the GDR.
4 Data are fully available to professionals and academics but are subject to special permission, and basic statistics are found in a widely available statistical yearbook, e.g. Poland.

Availability of foreign statistical information concerning crime in western countries is a separate problem for professionals and academics in eastern Europe; generally, such data are not easily available.

In eastern Europe, data concerning crime, except those published in official and widely available statistical publications, are always accompanied by a clause such as 'for service only' or 'for interior use only'. This means that they are covered by secrecy and are intended for use by bodies and institutions which represent the machinery of government which create an official and – in the view of the authorities – a desirable picture of criminality. Verification of the official view is not always possible due to the secrecy about sources of information.

Consequently this chapter inevitably has a number of inherent limitations. The comparison of the extent, structure and growth of crime in eastern Europe, if possible at all, must be approached with caution, and should not be used to draw far-reaching conclusions. Nevertheless, having recognised these limitations, comparative studies can usefully provide general indications and offer broad insights.

CRIME AND IDEOLOGY

I shall preface my remarks about crime in eastern Europe by presenting some views about the phenomenon of crime and the basic causes.

Marxist and Leninist ideology explains crime as a social phenomenon arising from private ownership and the consequent antagonism between social classes. Class contradictions achieve their ultimate expression in the capitalist system which pits labour against capital, and in which the wealth of the minority is in sharp contrast to the impoverishment of the working people. Simply stated, capitalism was thus understood to cause crime. The socialist system, on the other hand, as one of a social equality, was believed to abolish all antagonisms. The reasons for crime are abolished and subsequently crime itself, as socialism develops and is transformed into communism, should also disappear (Zwirbul 1976: 18ff).

This analysis was the starting-point of the socialist view of criminality, namely that the phenomenon of crime was based on the theory of 'capitalist relics'. According to this theory, crime exists in the socialist system only because of disadvantageous social and psychological factors and processes, such as anti-social and illegal traditions, customs and patterns descended from previous class antagonisms. Combat these 'relics' and the reasons for crime would be removed.

This theory, which was developed in Soviet writings as early as the 1930s, had an official binding force during the 'worship of the individual' period. Such an approach obviated the need for criminology as an independent branch of science. At that time criminology was regarded as a 'bourgeois branch of learning' which was quite superfluous in the socialist system (Kudriawcew *et al.* 1985: 138ff; Kuzniecowa 1976: 5ff). Subsequently the theory of 'relics' became binding also in other socialist states. In those states, as in the USSR, criminology could not develop.

However, in the course of time, it was observed that crime in fact had not disappeared and that 'capitalist relics' in the consciousness of society were perhaps not the only causes of crime. This realisation was understood, initially, to arise from disturbances in the development of socialism, as a result of which the authorities decided that some criminology research projects were necessary. These changes permitted the development of criminology in Poland and the USSR in the mid-1950s and in the GDR in the early 1960s.

In the present day, throughout much of eastern Europe, crime is understood to have multiple causes, including social, demographic, economic, psychological and biological factors. Individual authors, however, hold different opinions on specific criminological issues, but this is a phenomenon which is universal and certainly is not confined to eastern Europe countries. Indeed, it is now the case that in many socialist countries (particularly Poland and Hungary), crime problems are approached similarly to the way adopted by the capitalist countries. Crime is understood to be caused by broadly similar factors in countries of all political persuasions and is an inevitable product of the functioning of society.

The theory of 'relics', however, still has some currency, mainly in Soviet and the GDR's writings. It is stated from time to time that the development of socialism has, as yet, failed to resolve many important social problems, especially economic ones; this causes inequality between social classes, which is apparent in the fields of welfare, culture and consciousness. This status quo is regarded as a result of the has-been, capitalist social relations which are the direct cause of criminality, and which are an inevitable consequence of the transition from socialism into communism (Lekschas *et al.* 1983: 285ff; Oriechow 1976: 50ff; Schaarschmidt 1988: 97ff; Vagó 1976: 62ff).

POLAND, HUNGARY AND THE GDR: BACKGROUND

It is a commonly held view that crime is less widespread in socialist countries than in the capitalist ones and also that criminal behaviour is generally of a less serious nature. While levels of recorded crime provide only a partial reflection of reality, one should view official statistics, upon which my following comments are based, with extra caution not least because of the tumultuous changes which we are now experiencing throughout Europe (Schneider 1987: 268ff).

In this chapter data from three socialist European countries, Poland, Hungary and the GDR, are presented. First, each country's demography and legal systems will be described briefly.

Of the three, Poland is the largest, with a territory of more than 310,000 sq. km., a population of more than 37 million and a density of 119 inhabitants per sq. km. Population density is similar in Hungary; although it covers some 93,000 sq. km., Hungary has a population of less than 11 million. The GDR has a somewhat higher population density at 154 sq. km.; it covers some 100,000 sq. km., and has a population of more than 16 million.

In economic terms, the GDR is the most industrialised state. Its industry contributes about 70 per cent to the Gross National Product, which in recent years has been the ninth or tenth highest percentage in the world. Compared with the other two countries, the GDR is the most urbanised, with more than 76 per cent of its population concentrated in the urban areas. Hungary and Poland, however, have a more mixed economy of both industry and agriculture. The contribution of industry to the GNP in both countries is around 45 per cent, and of agriculture is about 20 per cent. In Poland, 60 per cent and in Hungary, 57 per cent of the population live in towns.

It should be borne in mind, however, that in Poland the 1980s were a period of far-reaching and unabated socio-political and economic crisis. The situation in Poland has therefore not been so stable as that in the other two and accordingly has been hardly comparable. Recent developments, however, could well change all that. The GDR and Hungary have been changing at such a dizzy pace that it is highly likely that criminologists a few years hence, will be able to plot changes in their crime rates coincident with their economic, political and social upheaval.

POLAND, HUNGARY AND THE GDR: LEGAL SYSTEMS

The legal systems of all socialist states, including those discussed here, are very similar to each other (Duft *et al.* 1981: 39ff; Fenyó 1975: 39ff; Frankowski 1987: 221ff).

In each of the countries considered in this chapter, the principle of legality is observed with respect to the prosecution of offenders. According to this principle, the public prosecutor or the police are obliged, having learnt about the alleged crime, to institute and conduct criminal proceedings; strictly speaking they have no discretion. This principle is clearly expressed in all penal codes of the socialist states. For example, the Polish Code of Criminal Procedure defines it as follows in Article 5 paragraph 1: 'The public prosecutor shall have the duty, *ex officio*, to institute proceedings with respect to an offence; the Civic Militia shall have the same duty'.

The principle of legality is however substantially limited by the so-called 'material concept of crime', which applies in the socialist states, but is unknown in the west. According to this concept, an offence is regarded as a criminal one if it involves a given degree of social danger. This is embodied in the penal codes of the socialist states, such as Article 1 of the Polish Penal Code, which states: 'Penal liability shall be incurred only by a person who commits a socially dangerous act prohibited under threat of a penalty by a law in force at the time of its commission'. Similarly Section 10 of the Hungarian Penal Code states: 'A criminal offence is an act, committed wilfully or – when the law also punishes a negligent commission – through negligence, that endangers society and is threatened by a penalty pursuant to the law'. This means that prosecution must be instituted only in the case of punishable behaviour which is dangerous to society to a sufficiently high degree, as defined by the law.

In all the three countries of this study, the notion of an offence is defined by the penal codes. Depending on their seriousness, criminal acts are defined as crimes (or felonies), or misdemeanours. Misdemeanours are punished the least severely, according to Article 5 of the Polish Penal Code, according to Section 11, part 1 of the Hungarian Penal Code and according to Paragraph 1 of the GDR's Penal Code. Petty offences or contraventions, on the other hand, are quite distinct from felonies, crimes and misdemeanours because they are regarded as acts which do not cause a sufficient degree of social danger for that behaviour to be considered a criminal one; as such they are not covered by penal codes and lie outside the penal courts' jurisdiction. They are also excluded from the criminal statistics.

CRIME STATISTICS

According to Polish statistical data, between 1980 and 1986, there were, on average, 458,759 crimes known to the police each year, that is 1,252 crimes per 100,000 people. In Hungary the respective figures were 157,539 and 1,477. In general, crime appears to be increasing. In Poland the number of crimes known to the police were 53 per cent higher in 1986 than in 1980 and the per capita increase was 42.8 per cent. In Hungary the absolute and per capita increases were 40.2 and 41.2 per cent respectively.

In the GDR, data concerning crimes known to the police are not available but it is possible to use data concerning convictions by courts. In 1980–6 there was an annual average of 121,152 convictions, that is 726 convictions per 100,000. Between 1980 and 1986, the absolute number of convictions fell by 12.3 per cent – a per capita reduction of 11.8 per cent.

In Poland, during the period in question, there were 142,310 convictions per year on average (333 per 100,000). Although the number of convictions fluctuated each year, it was slightly higher in 1986 than in 1980. Nevertheless, convictions per 100,000 appeared to be 8.7 per cent lower in 1986 than 1980 – a smaller fall than that in the GDR.

These figures indicate that in Poland one in four crimes known to the police resulted in a conviction: 1,252 crimes per 100,000 known to the police and 333 convictions. If we conjecture that in the GDR also, approximately one in every four crimes known to the police results in a conviction, we may guess that there are approximately four times as many crimes known to the police as convictions; we know that there were 726 convictions in the period in question so we may conjecture that in the GDR there were in the region of 2,732 crimes known to the police per 100,000. As statistics are not available in the GDR, we must resort to these calculations if we wish to try to compare like with like.

On the basis of these data cited above, we can guess that of the three socialist countries discussed here, Poland has the lowest level of crime, with Hungary being a very close second and crime seems to be the highest in the GDR. However, it would be unwise to extrapolate too much about this, in view of the speculative nature of the figures as discussed above.

THE NATURE OF CRIME

Crime in the countries discussed here is dominated by property crime. Between 1980 and 1986 in Poland, thefts were an average of 55.9 per cent of all crimes known to the police; this percentage was more or less stable. In Hungary the comparable figure was 45.7 per cent for 1986, this figure being approximately 50 per cent higher than the 1980 figure. This phenomenon is not easily explained with certainty, but it has coincided with economic changes during the 1980s including inflation and may also be connected with changes in recording practice.

In Poland between 1980 and 1986, the number of convictions for thefts was on average less than one-quarter of the number of thefts known to the police. If we speculate that a similar rate were also to apply to the GDR, thefts would amount to 41 per cent of all crimes known to the Republic's police. The difference between this figure and the published figure of 54.9 per cent of convictions being for thefts could be explained by the different rates of prosecution for different crimes by the police. There were 22 per cent more convictions for theft in 1986 than 1980. In Poland over the same period, an average of 36.7 per cent of convictions were for thefts and unlike in the GDR, this figure fell consistently, the 1986 rate being 26.8 per cent less than in 1980.

It thus appears to be the case that the GDR has the highest level of thefts of the three countries under consideration. However, it must be remembered that this presumption may be quite misleading because of the fact that the GDR authorities appear to convict more of those charged with theft than do the authorities in the other two countries.

In the socialist countries property offences are divided into two categories: offences against individual property and offences against social property. Penalties are much more severe for the latter category because of the special status of property owned by 'the people'. Offences against individual property are much more frequent, being on average more than two-thirds of all property offences.

As in western Europe, violent crime (which is defined the same as in western Europe) is very much in the minority, being, between 1980 and 1986, an average of 4.2 per cent and 5.6 per cent of all crime known to the police in Poland and Hungary respectively. Within these figures, robberies, rapes, manslaughters and assaults in Hungary were 0.9, 0.4, 0.3 and 4 per cent respectively. Equivalent figures for Poland were 1.5, 0.4, 0.1 and 2.2 per cent. It is apparent that significant differences for the two countries existed only for robberies and assaults. In both countries, the percentages of all crimes increased, being 38 per cent higher in Poland in 1986 than in 1980. Most of the increase in Poland arose from the considerable growth in the number of robberies, while the numbers of rapes, manslaughters and assaults dropped. In Hungary, the increase of violent offences was mainly attributable to the increased number of assaults.

As far as the GDR is concerned, an average of 10 per cent of convictions were for violent offences between 1980 and 1986, most of these being for assaults. In Poland 7.3 per cent of all convictions were for violent offences and, again, convictions for assaults dominate the statistics within the category of violent crime. If we assume that in the GDR, half of all violent offences known to the police result in convictions (as is the case in Poland), then we can conjecture that 4.4 per cent of offences known to the police in the GDR are of a violent nature.

EAST AND WEST: THE GDR AND THE FRG

Comparison of east and west Europe may be instructive and I shall therefore briefly compare the situations in the GDR and the FRG.

The FRG covers 248,000 sq. km. and has a population of over 60 million. The population density of 238 inhabitants per sq. km. is extremely high. The birth-rate in the FRG is very low and the population is in decline. It is a country which has been much affected by immigration, especially during the last decade.

As far as the economy goes, the FRG is a highly industrialised state, ranking fourth in the world in terms of total industrial production. Approximately 86 per cent of its population are concentrated in its urban areas.

In the legal system of the FRG (Herrmann 1987: 106ff), the principle of legality is observed with reference to the prosecution of offenders, but there are many concessions to the principle of discretion, which permit some leeway in the decision-making processes of the prosecuting authorities. They apply to some misdemeanours in the case of which the public prosecutor is free to decide whether to prosecute or not (see Sections 153–154d of the FRG's Code of Criminal Procedure). However, these concessions are not as important as in the socialist states and apply only to some misdemeanours in the case of which the public prosecutor is free to decide whether or not to prosecute.

Offences are divided – as in the socialist states – into two categories: crimes (felonies) and misdemeanours. Apart from offences, there are *Ordnungswidrigkeiten* (infringements) which are covered by a separate legal act; they are not subject to the jurisdiction of the penal courts and they are excluded from crime statistics.

In the years 1980–6, crimes known the police averaged 4,177,155 per year (6,808.1 per 100,000 population). Over the period, the former had increased by 14.4 per cent and the latter by 15.4 per cent. It would thus appear that both the total number of crimes known to the police, and the rate per 100,000, are much higher in the Federal Republic than in the three socialist states considered here although the precise situation in the GDR must remain conjecture because of the absence of police statistics.

Let us consider the structure of criminality. In the years 1980–6, thefts accounted for an annual average of 63.4 per cent per year of all crimes recorded by the police, this being somewhat larger than that recorded in the socialist countries. As in Poland, the rate remained more or less constant during the period in question. The equivalent rate of violent crimes was 5.2 per cent per year, being therefore higher than in Poland, but lower than in Hungary. As in the socialist countries, assaults were the dominant group within the category of violent offences. However, in the FRG, the proportion of assaults fell over the six years in question – by 9.1 per cent. At 0.1 per cent, the number of rapes in the FRG were clearly lower than in Poland and Hungary, as were robberies (0.7 per cent). On average, there were fewer cases of manslaughter in the FRG (0.1 per cent) and more assaults than in Poland.

So, if we compare the FRG with the three socialist countries some differences appear as far as recorded crime is concerned. However, the obvious perhaps needs to be stated. Crime in the FRG is no more representative of crime in the capitalist countries than is crime in the GDR, Poland or Hungary representative of crime in socialist countries.

What therefore should we make of all this statistical information? Is there really less crime in the socialist countries than in the capitalist ones, and does it manifest itself in different forms?

The opinion of scholars from the GDR is very consistent (Buchholz 1987: 61ff; Lekschas *et al.* 1983: 203ff) in so far as they believe that the level of criminality in the GDR is five to ten times lower than in the capitalist countries, particularly the FRG. According to them, such offences as thefts, frauds, manslaughter and robberies are very much less frequent in the socialist system. However, the problem is that these authors are comparing the GDR's conviction rate with the rate of crimes known to the police in the other countries. Like is not being compared with like. These types of data cannot of course be used for genuine comparison because they are measuring different things. On the basis of these statistical data, authors from the GDR contend that the GDR has one of the lowest crime levels in the world. However, we should recall the fact that the number of convictions per 100,000 is twice as high in the GDR as in Poland. In spite of this, it is interesting to note that Polish scholars do not claim that Poland is a particularly safe and crime-free country.

Also, the question of unreported crime should be considered. Numerous research projects carried out in the USA or in the countries of western Europe, such as the FRG, have proved that many criminal acts do not come to the attention of the authorities. Similar conclusions result from research projects conducted in Poland. Authors from the GDR still think that their 'hidden criminality' – the so-called 'dark figure' – is gradually decreasing because of close co-operation between the public and the police, and of their programme of crime prevention and control (Lekschas *et al.* 1983: 203). Unquestionably, in some socialist states, including the GDR, a very strict control is exerted by the state over its population. The police force acts more like an agent of state coercion than one which protects citizens against crime. There may be a general unwillingness therefore to report to the police, and crime may therefore be significantly under-reported; this of course is then reflected in the conviction rates. Also, the police are frequently unwilling to deal with the less serious crimes, which may nevertheless be very acute from the victim's viewpoint.

Co-operation between police and the public is therefore somewhat less effective than some authors from the GDR suggest. The official view of crime is much affected by the material concept of crime as mentioned above, that is by the degree of 'social danger' attributed to any criminal act. The critical decision about the degree of 'social danger' is decided by the prosecuting authorities which enjoy very wide discretionary powers in this regard. Obviously the decision of the prosecuting authorities significantly affects criminal statistics, as acts can be defined either as criminal or not, according to their evaluation.

Against the background of these observations, it is not astonishing to find reported in the comparative victimisation survey conducted in the FRG and Hungary in 1982, that not only were Hungarians more frequently victimised, but also they were less ready to report offences to the authorities than Germans in the FRG (Arnold and Korinek 1985: 65ff; Lammich and Nagy 1985: 176ff). The results of these surveys perhaps suggest that levels of crime do not vary from country to country as much as the official statistics would have us believe. Additional evidence of the imperfections of criminal statistics as a source of information, arises from the results of some research which indicates that the assumption of different levels of crime between particular countries, such as Poland, Yugoslavia, and Austria cannot be supported (Vodopiveč 1981: 1,048ff). Moreover, official statistics may be distorted by those who produce them. Indeed, from what we know of the corruption in the GDR before the revolution of 1989, it would be surprising if criminal statistics were totally reliable.

CONCLUSION

In general, the problems connected with crime in the socialist countries have not been adequately examined. Apart from the poverty of official statistical data, a special problem is the almost total lack of victimisation surveys. It is also to be borne in mind that criminality was (and to some extent still is) regarded as taboo, because of the ideological assumption of the 'vanishing' of crime under socialism.

Crime occurs under socialism for the same basic reasons as it occurs under capitalism. The hopes and aspirations of people are broadly similar under any system of government and the actual incidence of crime is intimately connected to the conditions in and the stability of society.

© 1991 Ewa Bienkowska

Chapter five

Women and crime in Europe

Frances Heidensohn

INTRODUCTION

Of all the developments in modern society changes in the perceived position of women have perhaps been the most remarked upon. Women in the majority of western nations have fewer than half the number of children their great-grandmothers did at the start of the twentieth century. Many now work in paid employment outside the home after, as well as before, marriage. Political and economic rights have been gained by women, often following considerable struggle, in most countries.

There is thus, at the end of the twentieth century, a climate of change in relation to women's roles. It is an international phenomenon with its source, like a rogue hurricane, in the USA, but prevailing winds have blown it across Europe. Issues related to women thus have a much higher profile today, both as policy matters and as subjects of analysis in the social sciences – which have themselves been much affected by these climatic changes. This then is the background to any study of women and crime in Europe today.

WOMEN AND CRIME

How then does the topic of women and crime fit into the concerns with sexual inequality and oppression? The links are not, at first, perhaps obvious. Crime is certainly a field of endeavour in which women could be said to have under-achieved. One of the earliest observations made when systematic criminal records were first kept was that convicted male offenders far exceeded females in number.

For much of the twentieth century, little or no work of substance was carried out on this topic. Only with the arrival of feminism, and especially 'feminist criminology' has this state of affairs been altered (Heidensohn 1985; ch. 8). Simply put, conceptual changes in the ways in which problems were perceived and analysed made it possible to address key issues in new and rewarding ways. Subjects which had been literally 'invisible' could be seriously addressed. As a result a new, much more socially and historically grounded study of the topic was instituted. Extensive accounts of these developments exist elsewhere (Heidensohn 1985; Naffine 1987). In brief, three major aspects of crime and women have become matters of interest and study. The first of these is the criminality of women, its trends and patterns, both as subject *per se* and in comparison with the criminality of men. Second is the criminology of women's crime, an area in which there have been significant developments and significant not merely to that topic. Finally there have been important and related changes to the agenda of concerns over crime and penal policy: that agenda has become a 'gendered' list. It is on these three aspects that I shall concentrate in this chapter.

Women and crime in Europe

One of the very few international comparisons of female crime groups western Europe and North America together as regions with similar levels of crime (Adler 1984). This is misleading. Although some accounts do add crime figures from different nations together to produce continental or hemispheric rates, this is a very dubious practice. Almost certainly, different things will be counted in each country. Adding European to North American rates also creates major distortions since the USA reports strikingly higher incidences of most offences than Canada (Hagan 1977) or Europe (Archer and Gartner 1984). There does appear to be something of a crime convergence between major European nations (van Dijk, Chapter 3 in this volume). However, since male offenders dominate all national crime figures, how far are there similarities in trends and patterns in female crime?

Only 10 per cent of the trouble?

An English commentator once observed that if men behaved like women the courts would be idle and the prisons empty. To a quite remarkable degree, crime is still an activity overwhelmingly dominated by men in all European countries. In France in 1986, of 809,059 persons *mises en cause* (i.e. dealt with in criminal proceedings) 81.27 per cent were male and 18.73 per cent female (*La Documentation Française* 1987). In England and Wales in the same year, 83 per cent of offenders found guilty or cautioned for indictable offences were male and 17 per cent female (Home Office 1986). In the Federal Republic of Germany in 1986, of those suspects proceeded against 79.5 per cent were male and 20.5 per cent female (Bundeskriminalamt 1987). (NB These figures do *not* of course measure the same stage of judicial proceedings.)

Reported figures for other nations differ somewhat, but do not vary greatly from this bench-mark. 'Irish criminal statistics show that the vast majority of those convicted are male' (Burke *et al.* 1981). In the Netherlands the female share of crime suspects has historically been about 10 per cent (Bruinsma *et al.* 1984) of persons charged by the police. For Norway in the same year, the ratio was 10.7 men to one woman (Central Bureau of Statistics of Norway 1988: 53) while in Italy convictions of women were 19 per cent of the total in the early 1980s. Scandinavian countries show similarly modest female contributions to the totals of crime at about 8 per cent for Finland (Antilla 1984) and Norway (Jensen 1984).

These are global figures and do not give a detailed or dynamic picture. Once we examine trends over time, type of offence, and so on, a more complex pattern is reflected. Nevertheless, the figures above fairly indicate the relatively modest contribution made by women.

Historically trends in female criminality have at several periods moved in opposite ways from those of men. Thus in England and Wales a higher proportion of those convicted in the early nineteenth century were female (Mannheim 1965) and this was also true of Denmark and Germany (Feest 1985) in the 1800s. In the twentieth century, whereas crime rates in general have risen, female criminality has stabilised, or at times fallen. In Austria, for instance, female criminality fell between 1953 and 1957 by 6 per cent whereas there was an overall rise of 10 per cent. During this period the proportion of convicted men to women rose from 5.2:1 to 7.4:1. In England and Wales the rates of convictions for indictable offences fell slightly during the 1950s. Stable and at times decreasing rates of female crime were described for Norway for various years during the 1970s and early 1980s (Jensen 1984). The most remarkable example, however, of decline in female criminality comes from Poland, where there was a 'steady and substantial decrease of female convictions in the 1960s and 1970s, a far more significant decrease than that experienced by men' (Plenska 1984). In fact, convictions of women fell 250 per cent between 1951 and 1977. Many of the nations which took part in the two World Wars saw relatively sharp rises in female crime and delinquency in these periods, nevertheless the relative rate of increase has often been slower for women than for men. Cario (1985) gives figures for France in Table 5.1.

Table 5.1 France: increases in recorded crime rates for men and women

	Population		*Crime*	
	Men	*Women*	*Men*	*Women*
1911	15,442,238	16,012,142	209,347	32,867
1982	21,462,215	21,681,923	647,507	54,350
Increase [a]	138	135	223	165

Note: [a] Where the figures for 1911 = 100
Source: Cario 1985

Such longer term analyses have proved important in the debates about the liberation causes – female – crime hypotheses which have been discussed since the 1970s. Surveying figures for 1935–75 in England and Wales, Smart not only observes the 'law-abiding' period of the 1950s mentioned above but also notes 'women offenders to be increasing at an overall faster rate than men' (Smart 1979; 54) except between 1965 and 1975 (although there are inconsistencies in the figures on violent offences [Austin 1981; Box and Hale 1983]). The 'new female offender' has been alleged to have become an internationally recognised phenomenon in the late twentieth century and to have sufficient impact to alter the direction of crime rates. Observations in various European countries suggest two kinds of patterns. In the first, typified by Finland and the Netherlands, female crime rates have risen, but not as fast as male rates. In others, notably France, the Federal Republic of Germany, and England and Wales, there is some evidence of relatively sharp increases in female rates. Comparing 1976 and 1986 there has clearly been a larger rise in female than male rates in the period (see Table 5.2). The Federal Republic of Germany has recorded some reduction in the numbers of suspected persons, but this has been much less in women than men (Table 5.3). For England and Wales, the faster rate of increase for women has already been observed. Between 1985 and 1986 there was an overall decline in numbers found guilty or cautioned 'mainly accounted for by males but the percentage decrease was equal for males and females' (Home Office 1986). The pattern for rates in relation to population was similar. What is striking about both the stable and the rising shares trends is that they both show that female crime rates move broadly in step with male crime rates (Box and Hale 1983: 43).

Table 5.2 France: proceedings against suspected persons (rate per 1,000 population at risk)

	Men	*Women*
1976	21.49	3.58
1986	30.04	6.44

Source: adapted from Ministry of the Interior 1987

Table 5.3 Germany: suspected persons (rate per 100,000 population at risk)

	Total	*Men*	*Women*
1982	2,934	4,979	1,105
1985	2,346	3,784	1,058
(% change)	-20%	-26%	-4.3%

Source: adapted from Bundeskriminalamt (ed.) 1985: Table 2.1.2, p. 13

Modest contributions?

Aggregating crime figures is a dubious task at best: the old adage about summing apples and pears applies forcefully to frauds and assaults. It is done to satisfy political and public demand for crime audits and accounts. More appropriate are breakdowns by types of offences: do women commit the same kinds of offences as men and as often and how similar are the patterns in different parts of Europe?

We have already seen that women commit comparatively little crime. Women, like men, are mainly accused and convicted of property offences. While definitions of crimes vary across judicial systems it is clear that the commonest crime committed by women is theft, very often in the form of shoplifting (Middendorf and Middendorf 1984; Feest 1985; Heidensohn 1985; Cario 1987). Fraud and forgery generally follow as the next commonest offences. It is important to stress that the offences most often committed by women are not necessarily those in which their *share* is greatest. Motoring offences are the largest category of all, but the female share is modest. After traffic violations and property crimes, drug-related offences have become more prevalent. Violent crimes are committed much less often by woman, although there have been increases among some younger age groups. Nevertheless, women do contribute to the tariff of all such crimes, including homicide.

The relative lack of female specialisation in crime is well illustrated in a summary table on four Scandinavian countries (Antilla 1984) showing no female participation rate above 50 per cent for any category of crime and none below 2 per cent. There are, of course, a few offences whose definition makes them specifically sex-linked in most jurisdictions. Rape is one obvious example: usually only men can be convicted of it, although women may be charged as accessories. Male but not usually female (except in Austria) homosexuality was widely criminalised in Europe until the 1960s and 1970s. Infanticide and self-induced abortion are female-only crimes. Most of these latter offences always appeared rarely in records and have now either been decriminalised or have minute rates.

Prostitution is one area where criminal laws may be said to be operated in a sex-related way. There is, however, great variety in definitions of offences related to prostitution and these are not always reported as fully as serious offences are. I have therefore included discussion of the topic in a later section (p. 67).

Most commentators agree on two additional attributes of female offenders. First, they commit fewer crimes and thus more of them are likely to be first offenders when arrested or tried than are men; second, very many fewer of them are professional criminals.

In summary, all European nations report a marked predominance of men in their criminal justice systems. Men figure as the most frequent suspected or convicted offenders both in total and for almost all offence and age groups. Women commit more crimes than they did earlier this century, but still far fewer than men, less often and less violently. These conclusions are drawn from administrative data from the criminal justice systems concerned. There have been attempts to find a larger iceberg-base of submerged female crime which would alter these findings. Various self-report studies and victim surveys have provided estimates of hidden female crime. They have not located excessive rates which would compensate for the major under-representation of women in official data. Most studies do find 'hidden' female crime, but they also find more 'dark-figure male' crime, so that the picture is modified, but not dramatically so. Dutch studies show more hidden offences by females under 18 (Bruinsma 1984) but do not alter adult ratios. One English study showed that males were more likely to indulge in undetected shoplifting and to steal more valuable goods (Buckle and Farrington 1984). Studies in Scandinavia have also revealed hidden female crime but not enough to raise the visible rates to male levels (Elmhorn 1969; Aromaa *et al.* 1970). The modest and marginal contribution made by women to offending has aroused criminological interest in the past twenty years and is discussed more fully below.

THE EXPERIENCES OF FEMALE OFFENDERS

It is perhaps not surprising that with such characteristics, very few female offenders are imprisoned in most European countries. Legal and penal policy changes have led to fluctuations and in general a decline in the numbers and the rate of female imprisonment in the twentieth century. In Norway and Finland (Jensen 1984; Antilla 1984) in the 1970s women comprised about 3 per cent or less of the prison population, for the Federal

Republic of Germany the figure was 3.7 per cent (Einsele 1981). In France there has been a decline in numbers of women in prison and the female share of the prison population since 1946. During the 1970s fewer than 1,000 women were imprisoned at any one time and they represented under 3 per cent of the total. By 1985 both figures had risen somewhat to 1,400 and 3.4 per cent respectively (Bibal *et al.* 1985: 76–8). Remarkably similar figures are reported for England and Wales (although it should be noted that a significant proportion of these are untried or unsentenced prisoners not subsequently sentenced to custody).

In smaller countries the numbers of women in custody are correspondingly tiny. In such instances, the lack of appropriate provision for them may not seem culpable. However, in practice, reports from almost all countries highlight problems and deficiencies in penal provision for women which sound remarkably similar notwithstanding very varied administrative systems. Three major themes emerge as concerns: problems due to the small, scattered numbers of women (the 'too few to count' argument), the double or triple deviance issue, and the question of paternalism.

Too few to count?

Women offenders do not, on the whole, benefit from their exclusive numbers. On the contrary, they suffer in several ways. Special provision is rarely made for them as they are so few: in England there is a specialised psychiatric prison, Grendon Underwood, for men, but no such provision is made for women. In Germany, because of its federal structure, 'young women are invariably housed in adult women's prisons – at best in specialized units' while young males can be separately housed (Einsele 1981: 6). Genders and Player (1986) report the same mixing in England and Wales. In centralised systems, the problem is usually one of few units widely scattered where women will be far from family, friends and home. Cario vividly describes the isolation of long-term prisoners in France in the sole Centre Penitentiaire Féminin which is in Rennes in Brittany (Cario 1985: 313ff). Osborough (1975) points out that girls sentenced to Borstal training (the predecessor to youth custody) in Northern Ireland used to have to go to Scotland to serve their sentences.

Some rungs of the sentencing tariff may not be provided for

women: detention centres were provided only briefly for young women in England and Wales. In Switzerland work and education centres have been provided for young men but not women (Einsele 1981: 62).

Double deviance

Personal accounts by convicted women (Carlen 1985; Heidensohn 1985) as well as an array of research findings insist that female offenders are perceived and treated as doubly deviant: they have transgressed society's rules by their crimes and by defying conventional norms of femininity. They thus feel peculiarly stigmatised and are also subject to particularly censorious and repressive treatment in the penal system.

Ida Koch (1983) has described the effects of this very vividly in her study of Denmark's co-educational prison. She points out that fellow male prisoners' censorious behaviour and attitudes were very much an additional punishment to women in this situation. The Dobashes in their study of Cornton Vale, the only prison for women in Scotland, noted that the inmates there felt 'a strong sense of shame and stigma' (Dobash *et al.* 1986: 187). Kersten in a comparative analysis of the treatment of young people in the Federal Republic of Germany concluded 'Girls in institutions have even less elbow-room as far as expectations of gender role conformity are posed [than boys]. In the event that they obviously "misbehave", the grasp of control becomes more forceful' (Kersten 1989: 143). An experimental integration of young male and female offenders at Eboli prison in Italy culminated in 'a full-scale revolt' in which girls took full and leading parts. The researchers reporting this suggest that this was due to the failure to address the conventional, feminine roles which the regime imposed on staff and on female inmates (Ferrari-Bravo and Arcidiacono 1989).

Gender roles and paternalism

There is notable congruence in numerous descriptions of institutions for women as explosive and dangerous places. While on the outside, women are generally perceived as the more conforming sex, inside prison they are said to be far more difficult to manage, more violent and more prone to need tranquillisers and other psychotropic drugs. Recent research and reports from several European countries have reassessed such accounts.

Institutions for women in the FRG, for example, are described as having 'an unrealistic institutional ethos, based on a moralistic assessment of behaviour' (Einsele 1981: 70). This finding is precisely paralleled in studies in women's prisons in England and Scotland. Women in these institutions were much more tightly controlled than in men's prisons, were reported for more trivial offences, and given less work and education than men (Carlen 1983; Dobash *et al.* 1986; Mandaraka-Sheppard 1986). What emerges very clearly from these researches is the oppressive, gender-stereotyped nature of the regimes in women's prisons:

> A female who does wrong even in the slightest detail must be made into a proper woman (who by definition does not do wrong) and this can be achieved through a therapeutic regime that seeks to reach even the most minute behaviour or motivation.
>
> (Dobash *et al.* 1986: 158)

Cario depicts an almost identical system at the CPF at Rennes: 'It perpetuates the values which our society attributes to the female role by the notable emphasis in the discipline system on obedience and submission and on educational activities of a traditionally feminine kind' (Cario 1985: 350 – my translation).

A further aspect of such paternalism reported from France concerns the system of conditional release. Reports on the characteristics qualifying women for this focus especially on submission, repentance, order, and hard work with a particular emphasis on family ties (Faugeron and Rivero 1982: 86–7).

In contrast, most institutional treatment for girls and women offers them far less than their male counterparts. In the FRG girls have 'a very narrow offering compared with boys' institutions, in the sector of work employment, leisure and adventure . . . this lack of offered pathways to social and economic independence' (Kersten 1989: 140).

The criminology of female crime

It is by definition very difficult for distinct criminal justice and social control systems to co-ordinate themselves and converge. That is indeed one of the major issues for such agencies in Europe after 1992. Cultural and intellectual barriers can often be more easily breached. It is clear from the account outlined above that there have been many comparable developments in female criminality across Europe. Concerns about women's penal treatment have converged even more closely. This is not just coincidence. In surveying the growing criminological literature on women it becomes clear that the new consciousness which I mentioned at the beginning of this chapter has had considerable impact on parts of European criminology.

The amount of work in this area has already grown considerably (Cain 1989). More significantly, however, than the growth in volume has been the direction in which discussions have run: they have for the most part taken a transatlantic turn.

Much of the key work in this field has been done in the USA and this has, inevitably perhaps, formed the foundations for most debates elsewhere, even when these have developed lives of their own. From a flourishing harvest I can pick out only a selection of choice products which illustrate richness as well as both convergence and diversity. This is not a comprehensive choice but is, I hope, reasonably representative.

Rates and rises

Only one approach to female criminality has ever managed to penetrate popular consciousness and thus become instantly recognisable. This is the 'liberation causes female crime' argument proffered by Adler (1975) and in modified form by Simon (1975). Adler endeavoured to explain allegedly rapid rises in female crime rates by linking them to the women's movement. She argued that the latter had spawned a new kind of female criminal who was tough, aggressive and violent, preferring to rob banks rather than to mind babies. Adler's statistical analyses as well as her arguments have been extensively criticised and her thesis refuted (Smart 1979). What is instructive to note is the way in which discussions about women's crimes in Europe have centred round this hypothesis.

That British studies should do so is perhaps not surprising, given the common language and close cultural and academic ties. There were also, as in most of Europe, certain phenomena to explain, notably faster rises in female than male crime. Feminist criminology had had, however, an early and distinctive start in

Britain (Heidensohn 1968; Smart 1977; Gelsthorpe and Morris 1988) and while engaging somewhat in the rates, rises and new female criminal debates, other issues have also been on the main agenda. One of the most important has been that of altering the assumptions of mainstream criminology to see that sex and gender are no longer neglected issues (Carlen and Worrall 1987; Heidensohn 1987). In the long run the most important result of studying female crime may lie in what we learn about all, especially male, crime.

Many papers on female crime in Europe take on the task of refuting Adler's relevance to their territory (Feest 1985) including several in a volume edited by her (Jensen 1984). In some areas this has also involved tackling the one distinctive manifestation of female criminality in the twentieth century: the female terrorist. Acts of political terrorism featured particularly in Europe in the 1970s and 1980s, although they have a long history. In Ireland, Italy, the FRG, France and Britain there were bombings, kidnaps, assassinations and sieges. The ideologies claimed by the perpetrators were very diverse and spanned from far left to far right yet nearly all had a significant representation of women amongst active members and leaders. Some of these, especially in the FRG, became very well known. Attempts to explain the female terrorist have been rather limited, at best highly individualist descriptions of cases. One German commentator notes the sexism of such accounts which 'seem incapable of seeing women as human beings who can be violent criminals or even politically active'. She points out that no female terrorist has ever claimed allegiance to the women's movement (Einsele 1981: 60).

Marginalisation and female crime

While the debate on liberation and crime can be seen as a damaging diversion, in refuting the arguments criminologists have had to explore other explanations of features of female crime. In doing so they have helped to bury another moribund argument, concerning the sexualisation of female criminality. It can sometimes seem to the experienced student of this subject that someone is always trying to glamorise it. In the earlier version of this transformation, crime-prone Cinderella's behaviour was attributed to her hormones, the stages of her generative cycle, her sexuality or lack of it. In the emancipation era, power and liberty replaced sex as causative factors. Both these interpretations distort by glossing over the observed characteristics of female offenders.

Studies of imprisoned women in Britain show their poverty, lack of education, and of skills or work record. Many have children, few have stable partners and most report a lack of choice, autonomy and order in their lives (Genders and Player 1986; Carlen 1983, 1985). Research and the activities of prostitute women themselves have re-presented prostitution as an economic, not a primarily sexual activity, through which women earn cash to keep themselves and their families (McCleod 1982; Heidensohn 1985). Several contributors to a symposium on girls and social control in Europe note the importance of economic factors in determining both their deviant behaviour and, during the recession of the 1980s, the 'increasingly punitive response by our European penal systems' (Cain 1989).

Another version of this approach has developed in Scandinavia. In an influential article, Cecilie Høigård analysed Norwegian figures on female crime and concluded that explanations related to liberation changes in gender patterns or the new opportunities for women to commit crime at work were not adequate. Instead she put forward a theory of 'expulsion', arguing that the relationship between gender and class has altered in modern society so that gender has become more important. Women offenders are recruited from those at the bottom and margins of society (Høigård and Snare 1983; Folgesvold and Dullum 1988). Gender analysis has also characterised a number of studies of young delinquent women and girls involved in a variety of deviant activities (Cain 1989).

Chivalry

One debating topic set by American criminology has been widely debated across Europe. This is the 'chivalry' debate. Criminologists in the past often asserted that the police and the courts favoured women, treating them more leniently than men. Such assertions were usually based on lower female crime rates and even lower imprisonment rates. The consensus from a series of West German studies seems to be that 'the theory that the crime prevention authorities treat women better and that women are less thoroughly investigated more frequently released and less harshly judged can be taken as disproved' (Steffen 1983: 12). Similar findings are reported from Austria (Einsele 1981).

In one French study comparing the treatment of male and female offenders, the chivalry hypothesis is only one of the possible explanations considered. The authors nevertheless acknowledge its importance as a focus of discussion. They observe that there is some differential treatment and ambiguity in the treatment of women offenders in France (Faugeron and Rivero 1982). A number of empirical studies in Britain have been reviewed by Lorna Smith (1988), who highlights some problems of definition: does *equal treatment* for men and women mean the *same treatment*? At least one British researcher found that women were more likely to be treated leniently by the courts than men (Allen 1987). Europeans have adapted and developed American ideas for their own use in analysing female crime. The adaptations have generally proved fruitful and successful, although it is often clear that the framework of the debate is what the French call 'anglo saxon'. There are also of course many distinctive local concerns of which discussions about women and social control are perhaps the most notable.

The new crime agenda

In Europe and in most developed countries there is a new agenda for social control agencies and for the general public. Priorities for policing have been redefined and policies and practices altered. There are a number of common characteristics on this agenda: these include an emphasis on crime control, a focus on the victims of crime and a redefinition of a number of crimes as having gender links. While all three are to some extent linked, it is the third point which has most salience for our purposes.

With the world-wide growth of victim movements (Shapland *et al.* 1985), the role and position of crime victims has been increasingly acknowledged and supported. Fear of crime is now recognised as a major inhibitor of freedom, especially in some inner city areas. One aspect of this has been recognition of significant gender differences. Thanks to a series of feminist and related studies, it is clear that while young men are often the victims (and the perpetrators) of street violence, women are the main victims of domestic violence, child sex abuse and rape (Stanko 1984). Most

European countries have responded by providing shelters and support for victims and by altering policing priorities. These are small steps so far, but they are Europe-wide, even if they have their own forms in each nation, and they represent the internationalising of certain concepts of social problems. There are doubts about how these concerns may be manipulated but not about the importance of the issues.

CONCLUSIONS AND PROPOSALS

Patterns and trends of female crime in Europe do seem to parallel each other very closely. Low recorded levels, modest crimes, little recidivism and no specialisation characterise most nations. Approaches to the understanding of these issues are also linked by common themes, and these often have an American or Anglo-American tone. These are, however, the characteristics of nation states, not of the whole continent. Is there a truly European dimension to female crime?

Several crime trends do cross national barriers very readily, most notably, in this field, substance abuse and prostitution. Women's contribution to the first is growing. Prostitution also seems to be attracting more participants not only because of the number of drug users who need to finance their habit, but also, with high unemployment and high divorce rates, because more women are forced to sell their bodies to support their families.

It is interesting to observe that several historic Europe-wide 'crime' waves have involved women. The persecution of witches in the sixteenth to eighteenth centuries killed off large numbers of women, especially in Scotland and Germany (Larner 1981). In the nineteenth century there was an international movement to outlaw prostitution and its state regulation. It was founded in Britain and spread to France, Germany and Switzerland (Petrie 1971). More recently, women have been strongly associated with terrorism in Europe. Can we draw any conclusions from these historical accounts? From the first and last perhaps, to be wary of moral panics which can often involve women and to their detriment. From the second we may conclude that power may sometimes be successfully used by women to help each other. The International Association cut across national and class barriers to achieve its aims.

Proposals

This chapter represents one attempt to make comparisons across Europe. In order to achieve future results in this field two aims have to be achieved. First, the key message of feminist criminology must strike home: acknowledge gender everywhere. There are still too many sets of data without sex breakdowns. Research studies are still published which ignore or omit females or, worse still, are unclear on the point. Second, more comparative data need to be made available and in usable form. This is as true of research findings as of official figures. It is a great pity that many studies are not more widely available, either translated into a major language or in fully published form. My impression in working on this chapter has been of dealing with a samizdat subculture.

Comparative study has much to offer any criminologist: cultural differences can provide instant control groups (as well as complications). For policy-makers there is the chance to learn about other solutions to the same problems – and failed experiments. Comparisons involving women are even fewer than those dealing with men. They should, I believe, be encouraged not only for the obvious general reasons, but also for certain specific ones.

First, the crime agenda has changed. Women played some part in achieving that change and are involved in monitoring many of the new agenda's projects. They can no longer be ignored in this nor in other areas. There are many lessons to be learnt about topics as diverse as child sex abuse and the diversion of women in the criminal justice system. Finally, there is an important possible gain for work on crime in general. As I have tried to demonstrate, there is remarkable consistency in European crime patterns. Across a range of cultures, climates and histories women conform and men commit crime. If crime is a major European problem, we must surely be able to learn something from studying this Europe-wide situation.

© 1991 Frances Heidensohn

ACKNOWLEDGEMENTS

Many people helped me in the preparation of this chapter by

sending me tables, reports and research studies. I am most grateful to Robert Cario, Jane Dullum, Lionel Fontagné, Claude Faugeron, Brit Nora Folgesvold, Ida Koch, Arno Pilgram, Renée Van Swaningen and Hartmut Weber.

Chapter six

Drugs, crime and law enforcement

Some issues for Europe[1]

Nick Dorn and Nigel South

INTRODUCTION

In this chapter we shall provide a rapid over-view of recent developments in European drug use,[2] approaches to its control and related issues such as responses to the spread of HIV. We shall briefly review the debates over the nature of any link between drug use and acquisitive or violent crime and question the dominant image of drug markets as monopolistic. We shall also review the development and uptake of domestic legislation and bilateral agreements aimed to facilitate the confiscation of the assets of drug-traffickers. We shall offer some observations on the relevance of the European Single Market for drug use, control and policy, concluding with some observations on existing arenas of co-operation and on the prospects for mutual assistance between law-enforcement agencies in relation to intelligence sharing and operational matters.

DRUG USE IN EUROPE: THE SHIFT TO COCAINE

In the late twentieth century most European countries share an awareness of the growth of illicit drug use and related problems. Historically there has been a shift from the serious concern about the relatively uncommon and localised use of those drugs called 'soft' in the 1960s, to a more widespread pattern of opiate and multi-drug use today.

The situation in the late 1980s was quite different from that of the 1960s when, in Europe at least, illegal drugs were more talked about than taken, more *represented* than consumed. At that time drugs were linked in popular, academic and official accounts to new youth cultures frequently seen as expressing some kind of liberationist or 'counter-cultural' philosophy. The drugs which received most attention were cannabis and to a lesser extent LSD and amphetamine (speed). Regional variations in official reporting of drug use offer a patchy picture (cf. Hartnoll 1986) and may partially explain the different degrees of concern which 'drugs' elicited in different countries in the 1960s, although evidently cultural factors played a significant role too. Since the mid-1970s, counter-cultural aspirations have largely faded and a different but more pervasive pattern of drug involvements has developed.

Of particular significance from a European perspective has been the recognition of widespread illicit drug use in countries with little past history of such problems – countries such as Italy, Spain, Poland and Greece – at the same time as there has been a dramatic rise in the availability and use of heroin across the European continent (Hartnoll 1986: 15). From the mid-1970s for example, the supply of heroin from south-west Asia (the 'Golden Crescent') to the Federal Republic of Germany rose sharply; in the UK, south-west Asian heroin developed a market later in the decade (around 1979) after a wave of refugees entered the country following the fall of the Shah of Iran. Elsewhere, as in the Netherlands and France, heroin from south-east Asia (the 'Golden Triangle') had traditionally been available. Heroin from the same source was also available in Italy but in the late 1970s use of the drug grew considerably with the addition of south-west Asian heroin and also Sicilian heroin (Hartnoll 1986: 15). The latter source is relatively new with a recent Interpol report recording that 'in 1984, the first major opium poppy cultivation operation in [continental] Europe was reported when 7,500 plants were discovered in Italy' (Interpol 1986: 47).

Problems related to the use of stimulants are also common throughout Europe and in some places, such as Sweden, are the predominant concern. The high profile recently given to cocaine and crack follows repeated claims throughout the 1980s by US enforcement sources that the North American cocaine market is saturated and that Europe will soon be overwhelmed by the diverted surplus. However, a cautious appraisal of the limited evidence available would be advisable. The proposition that demand in North America is saturated is questionable while estimates of the size of the market for cocaine and crack in Europe are highly variable. For example, while Lewis (1989) observes that

'London, Rome and Amsterdam are cities with established cocaine markets, that are also points of transit for shipments destined for other European centres', he also acknowledges that the cocaine market 'varies in size from city to city and from country to country. Individual consumption tends to be intermittent, which creates difficulties in estimating the extent of actual demand' (Lewis 1989: 47–8).

Law-enforcement agencies and the media are currently much exercised by the threat of crack, with considerable pressure from the US Drugs Enforcement Administration (DEA) for Britain to recognise this as *the* drug problem of the future. Crack, a form of 'free-base' cocaine, may be made in a quite simple process from the more commonly available cocaine hydrochloride; the availability of cocaine itself has risen in most parts of Europe during the 1980s. By 1988, across Europe as a whole, seizures of cocaine were greater on a kilogram basis than seizures of heroin.[3] It is quite possible that the increase in cocaine seizures reflects the growth of the cocaine trade in Europe to some extent, although increasing resources targeted on this drug may have generated some of the increase in seizures. As far as free-base versions of cocaine were concerned, there were very few seizures in Europe in the late 1980s. In Britain, for which we have up-to-date figures, there were twenty-three seizures of crack in the first half of 1989, a rate of seizure that is about double that of 1988. Some of the increase in recorded seizures of crack in Britain may be due to strong directives to the police to target this drug and to notify every seizure to the National Drugs Intelligence Unit immediately, but there does appear to have been a real increase in the underlying pool of availability of crack following extensive publicity in the first half of 1989. This was generated by a series of speeches given by a visiting DEA agent to British police officers, a number of ministerial statements, and widespread media accounts of a sensational new drug and how to make it (*Druglink* 1989a). The obvious danger of such publicity lies in the way that it alerts and attracts potential users and dealers.

Opinions vary about the potential for a pan-European crack or cocaine problem to (1) spread widely and (2) take the same social form as it apparently takes in some US cities. In Amsterdam, for example, one respected commentator reports that 'crack-cocaine as a ready-to-use product was marketed in the Netherlands as early as 1973, but it did not catch on and is hardly seen on the streets since' (van Vliet 1989: 28).

The future of cocaine in Europe remains to be experienced. It is worth while bearing in mind, however, that cocaine-related problems in Europe so far are of a much smaller magnitude than problems related to other drugs. Throughout Europe, heroin and amphetamine should be noted as sources of concern, while cannabis is the most commonly taken drug, albeit in some countries partially decriminalised for possession and use of small amounts. As far as harmfulness is concerned, it is the sharing of injection equipment and the practice of unsafe sex between drug/alcohol users and their partners that is the most serious problem, for reasons that we now discuss.

DRUGS AND HIV: THE UNCLAIMED PROBLEM

Whether one is talking about heroin, amphetamine or cocaine, the practice of injection amongst some social groups gives rise to the public health issue of how to prevent the spread of HIV, the AIDS virus, between people who are sharing syringes who may pass on the virus to others and to non-injecting sexual partners. This is a truly international problem with no respect for borders – and it is also one which is having its impact on thinking about how to reconcile law-enforcement policy with policy about the provision of drug services, such as syringe exchange schemes. In some countries such a reconciliation may be easier to accomplish than in others. In the Netherlands, for example, syringe exchange programs for intravenous drug users are viewed as 'well-considered tools meant to implement the Netherlands' general and specific social, health and judicial policies' (van Vliet 1989: 28).

In Switzerland, by contrast, the tension between differing law enforcement and public health goals has been heightened by the introduction of such schemes. Switzerland has a very high incidence of HIV and Zurich is recognised as having the highest number of drug users in the country. The city council and medical services have therefore promoted a policy which aims to prevent further transmission of HIV. An unofficially decriminalised zone was established in a city park where small-scale dealing and use has been tolerated and a syringe exchange scheme successfully established. To the city police force, however, the park area has become a magnet for drug users from

> all over Switzerland and Europe, with an inevitable rise in crime . . . The contradiction between the strategies of police and city council is evident: 'It's politically very hard to carry out a raid when soup is just being dished out' (second-in-command, Zurich Police).
>
> (*Police Review* 1989c: 1,656)

The situation in Britain may fall somewhere between the harmonious integration of policies so frequently claimed as the Netherlands approach and the tensions displayed in the Swiss example. A large number of syringe exchange schemes have been established with modest successes (Stimson *et al.* 1988), and the idea of reducing the *harm* that can follow from drug use rather than solely focusing on reduction of use has also been accepted in government thinking (Advisory Council on the Misuse of Drugs 1984). The Department of Health, for example, has recently funded local drugs and HIV information campaigns, one of which involved the distribution of a leaflet for injectors giving 'up-front advice on injecting that would have been unthinkable in a government-funded publication before HIV legitimised harm reduction' (*Druglink* 1989b: 11).

None the less, in terms of the balance of emphasis in government policy and response to drugs in Britain, it is law enforcement which has formed the central thrust of the government's strategy (Home Office 1985a), not health. Indeed, the high-level Cabinet Committee overseeing AIDS policy was abolished in the summer of 1989, signalling a downward momentum for HIV and AIDS as an issue of high political priority. Increasingly in Britain, and indeed elsewhere in Europe, the balance of political priorities reflects a concern not only with the illegality of possession and use of drugs, but also about the profits that are generated by drug-trafficking (Dorn and South 1990a) and about the relationships between drug use and dealing and other forms of crime.

DRUGS AND CRIME: COMPETING HYPOTHESES

There are two principal (and one hybrid) explanations of any relationship between illegal drug use and crime (other than straightforward possession or use where in different countries these are illegal acts in themselves). In summary, these are first, that drug use leads to crime; second, that involvement in crime leads to drug use; third, that both crime and drug use are the results of some other factors (Research Triangle Institute 1976: 54). Despite the popularly dominating image being that drug use causes crime, the evidence from the available literature has always been far less clear. As one major US review put it

> There is no evidence that opiates are a cause of crime in the sense that they invariably lead to criminality, but there is no doubt that among those addicts with a delinquent lifestyle drug use is part and parcel of their other activities, crime included.
>
> (Blum 1967)

Other factors that may be important features of a drug-using life-style include involvement in the informal/irregular 'street' economy where drugs may be just one commodity among many that are bought and sold. Working, hustling and committing petty crimes in this 'street' environment may be the context in which someone is introduced to heroin, for example, perhaps as a reward or celebration after a successful job. Hence involvement in crime can lead to involvement with drugs rather than vice versa (Auld *et al.* 1986).

The investigation of the dynamics of such involvements has largely been undertaken in North America and generalisations to the drug-using subcultures of individual European nations or to Europe as a whole might be unjustified. But there are certainly pointers in some recent British studies that indicate that the conventionally assumed direction of causality linking drugs to crime is questionable and that the crime–drugs relationship is far more complex. There is a need for further European studies (perhaps comparative across several countries) on this question, and a need for the publicising and more effective dissemination of the limited research findings that we do have.[4]

DRUGS AND TRAFFICKING: PATTERNS OF DISTRIBUTION

As there have been challenges to the common perception of the 'drugs causes crime' connection, so have traditional economistic models of supply and demand as explanations of drug use and consumption recently been questioned. In these models the dynamic force responsible for expanding the market in drugs may be 'organised crime' in monopolistic forms (supply-push model), or 'consumer demand' for drugs (where demand is assumed to be caused by individual psychopathology, social ignorance or structural unemployment) or both supply-push and demand-pull.

However, greater awareness of a much broader range of participants in drug markets has led to recognition of the vital importance of the distribution channels *between* consumers (demand) and producers (supply). Three factors have contributed to this. First, in Britain, as elsewhere in Europe, this recognition follows from the spread of drug distribution in the 1980s beyond those areas in which it was traditionally focused, and across Europe into countries that previously had very little in the way of illegal drug problems. Second, law-enforcement agencies throughout Europe have been paying more attention to anti-distribution strategies. At the same time, economically informed research (principally conducted in the USA) has drawn attention to the complexity of drug markets, their personnel and economic composition (e.g. B. Johnson *et al.* 1985). Third, research which challenges stereotypes of monopolistic organised crime has also been influential in suggesting the need to re-think the structure of drug markets (e.g. Reuter 1983).

If the old linear conception of monopolistic supplier to point of demand is so much of an over-simplification, then what would a more adequate picture of drug markets be? While not denying the significance of groups such as the Sicilian *Mafia* or Neapolitan *Camorra* (Lewis 1989: 40), we believe that a more sophisticated model of drug markets can be drawn than that normally presented in popular media. From fieldwork and the international literature, it is possible to identify at least seven types of small to large-scale enterprises involved in illicit drugs distribution (cf. Dorn and South 1990b). But recognition of this diversity of participants in drug markets also has implications for our understanding of how law enforcement works – for the two are locked in an interactive and mutually influencing relationship. As a recent Interpol report described this interaction:

> Both traffickers and drug law enforcement services rely on flexibility for their successes. The traffickers change their routes, their couriers and their methods of concealment as soon as one or the other becomes exposed. Equally, law enforcement agencies have to respond to and indeed anticipate new trends,

given that the chances of success are, at the present time, heavily biased in favour of the traffickers.

(Interpol 1987: 17)

New trends and developments in drug markets are almost certain. They may come from changes in the conditions prevailing in the North American market, or as the result of President Bush's push for stiffer anti-trafficking measures in South America or as a consequence of the easing of internal movement in Europe after 1991/2. Even more than in the past, a more accurate conception of the diverse and polymorphous nature of drug markets will be a necessary prerequisite for the future success of law-enforcement strategies and the policies that affect them.

DRUGS AND 1992: DISTINGUISHING THE FLOWS OF DRUGS AND THE FLOWS OF MONEY

We can only speculate about any impact that the 1992 lowering of trade and customs barriers will have on drug distribution and related crime. In recent interviews that we have conducted, a number of British police and customs officers have advanced quite different views of the likely consequences.[5] Essentially these are that either the new development will make no difference or that its impact will be profound.

The former position is based on the belief that trade and customs barriers within the European Community are already relaxed and that the amount of commercial, business and tourist travel between countries is so high as to make effective customs inspection very difficult as things are. The increased, and inevitably increasing, use of sealed containers to move cargo internationally by truck or boat also makes it virtually impossible to check all import and export movements. Given all these current conditions, some would argue that 1992 will make little difference to levels of drug distribution. Those who express more concern may agree with this latter proposition, but would argue that what they fear is that the easing of business and general financial transactions will facilitate the movement of the *profits* of drug distribution from one legal jurisdiction to another.

There is little in the way of empirical evidence that we can point to in order to gauge which of the views on the consequences of the raising of the barriers is the more realistic. Interpol (1986: 48) noted that in July 1984 border controls between France and the Federal Republic of Germany were relaxed 'considerably': 'this measure, adopted as part of the "open border" policy of the EEC, makes it possible for people to cross between these two countries without undergoing systematic checks, unless special instructions are issued'. The result with regard to drug-trafficking across the border is unhelpful and unclear because 'in the month that followed there was a significant increase in the number of persons arrested for narcotics trafficking although this upward trend has not yet been confirmed' (Interpol 1986: 48).

The Schengen Treaty, signed in 1985 by France, the FRG, Belgium, Luxembourg and the Netherlands, initially foresaw working toward the abolition of frontier controls at the common borders of its signatories by the end of 1990 – a target which has now been deferred to 1992 (Jenkins 1989: 12). Yet this precursor to 1992 has attracted little attention and does not seem to be cited by any commentators as a factor in the expansion of drug distribution in Europe in the late 1980s.

On balance, it would seem likely that some drug-dealing entrepreneurs will attempt to take whatever advantage that they can of more open trade channels after 1992. However, whether this will make a considerable difference to the drug distribution system is more debatable. Certainly, with respect to Britain, the government is expecting that HM Customs and Excise will continue to follow similar border control procedures to those currently in operation and one of its major justifications for doing so is concern over the importance of drugs. As Mr Douglas Hogg, Under Secretary at the Home Office, told the House of Commons in June 1989:

> the Home Secretary has made it quite plain by treaty and by statute that we have retained the right to maintain at the ports of entry such controls as we deem necessary to prevent the importation of drugs and other criminal articles.
>
> (*Hansard* 1989: 522–3)

Hence in respect of UK border controls at least, 1992 will see little change.

What is certain is that drug distribution may be less risky if it is easier to move the profits from one country to another, beyond the reach of domestic law-enforcement agencies. Police and customs officers who have been developing investigative strategies to trace and seize such profits are concerned that the absence of agreements between EC countries over financial investigations and seizure of assets will mean that large sums will 'disappear'.

Progress in negotiating such agreements has been slow despite enthusiastic encouragement from Britain and the USA and the recommendations of the June 1987 United Nations International Conference on Drug Abuse and Illicit Trafficking. These recommendations included passing legislation to enable the forfeiture of the assets and equipment of drug-traffickers and to improve extradition procedures. The recommendation that control over international movement of freight be tightened evidently faces some practical problems as 1992 nears.

It appears that one of the problems slowing the process of negotiating the international agreements is that different countries want different kinds of treaties. The UK government favours bilateral agreements between countries and, by mid-1989, had signed such treaties with two European countries, Spain and Switzerland, and was in negotiation with two others, France and the Federal Republic of Germany.[6] Some other countries prefer multilateral agreements, while others have expressed a wish to see the subject matter of the agreements broadened to cover more than just profits generated by drug crime. Such agreements *will* eventually emerge, building upon and linking up legislation that already exists in some countries, such as Britain (where the Drug Trafficking Offences Act 1986 has provided new tools for financial investigations as well as new penalties: Dorn and South 1990a), the Federal Republic of Germany (where drug-related asset seizure legislation has just been introduced and anti-money laundering legislation is being developed: *Police Review* 1989b: 1,509), and Italy (where controls on bank deposits and other transactions have recently been introduced to detect and deter the laundering of drug profits: Sheridan 1989). The questions remain of when such international agreements may be established and working, and how effective they may be.

CONCLUSION: A EUROPEAN DRUG ENFORCEMENT ADMINISTRATION?

There are already in existence a large number of organisations and groups which deliberate on drug problems and responses in Europe. These include the nineteen-nation Pompidou Group, established in 1971 with a remit to co-ordinate responses to drug-trafficking, but which has also considered European treatment policy and research needs: the twelve-nation TREVI Group which has a broader brief, including drug-trafficking along with terrorism and similar issues, and which acts as a clearing house passing on intelligence and policy briefings between participating agencies; and the newly formed (1988) European Regional Secretariat of Interpol (Wallace 1989). In addition, there are three Directorates within the European Community administration which have been involved in fostering collaborative work between different countries on drugs issues, while the European Parliament has also generated working parties and carried out a Committee of Enquiry on the subject (Hartnoll 1989: 39). More recently, in July 1989, the so-called Group of Seven nations met in Paris with drugs on their agenda, one outcome being support for Mrs Thatcher's proposal for a meeting in London in 1990 for further discussions of possible ways to reduce the demand for and trafficking in drugs.

To the fore in nearly all these initiatives has been consideration of law-enforcement and legislative responses to drug use and drug-trafficking. It is in this area then that we can most confidently expect to see new developments in the approach to, and after, 1992. For the time being, European law-enforcement agencies concerned with illegal drugs interdiction are faced by two new challenges. First, how to best employ the new techniques of financial investigations and drug profit confiscation procedures that are being opened up to them, and second, how to build up opportunities for mutual co-operation between European drug investigators.

In order to pursue both these goals more efficiently, we may in the future perhaps see the development of a European 'Drugs Enforcement Administration' on the US model. Alternatively this might have a broader brief and also cover terrorist activities, in certain respects being an operational reflection of the TREVI Group.

The development of a more intelligence-oriented drugs agency, a pan-European version of Britain's highly regarded National Drugs Intelligence Unit, would be another possibility. Such an agency was mooted in April 1989 by Britain's then Home Secretary, Mr Douglas Hurd, who told Association of Chief Police Officers' (ACPOs) National Drug Conference that 'there should be a unit to develop intelligence and promote closer co-operation on a European basis' (*Police Review* 1989a: 846). Mr Hurd said that he had already suggested this idea to European colleagues, but that it was as yet too early to give details (*Police Review* 1989a: 846).

With regard to this latter possibility, we may note, perhaps with some caution, that among the goals of the Schengen Treaty partners is a proposal to develop a comprehensive information system. One draft description of this system states that 'in order to compensate for the disappearance of internal frontier controls, an exchange of information between police and security authorities is indispensable' (Jenkins 1989: 12). In some form or another, such a proposal will no doubt be incorporated into future European Community administrative plans.

By 1989, across Europe, increased information exchange, closer co-operation between law-enforcement agencies and more legislation and treaties facilitating mutual assistance in financial and other investigations, were all developments already with us. In the 1990s they will be built upon quite considerably.

Such enhanced co-operation and possible organisational developments could be important strategic innovations. On the other hand they may also be accompanied by some measures that will seem unpalatable. There is still considerable need for research and informed debate on the kinds of responses to problems of drugs and crime that will be appropriate for Europe in the 1990s.

© 1991 Nick Dorn and Nigel South

Chapter seven

Ethnic minorities

Crime and criminal justice in Europe

Hans-Jörg Albrecht

INTRODUCTION

Deep concern for the problem of foreign and ethnic minorities in relation to criminal justice exists today in virtually all European countries. Everywhere, substantial numbers of people with an ethnic background differing from that of the society at large have settled down. It seems obvious that the concept of the *Gastarbeiter* (migrant worker or guest-worker), which has been used in some countries to avoid the effects and costs of immigration and permanent settlement, is no longer appropriate to the current situation of ethnic minorities. Those *Gastarbeiter* obviously did not come to the host country for short periods of time in order to supply labour but stayed on a permanent basis and most importantly, brought their families with them. Consequently about 60 per cent of foreigners living in the Federal Republic of Germany (FRG) have done so for more than ten years. *Gastarbeiter*, according to the official policies of, for example, Austria, FRG, Switzerland and France, should have helped to meet short- and middle-term demand for personnel during the economic boom of the 1960s. Their legal status (as far as other than EC citizens are concerned) is in some respects different from that of nationals (for a complete summary covering the European Community see Just and Groth 1985: 82–111). For example, they are not allowed to vote or to be elected, they may not hold positions in the Civil Service and, most importantly, in general, they have no permanent right of residence but have only limited permits. Although most countries in Europe have set up severe restrictions to immigration in the 1980s and some have implemented programmes designed to provide incentives for foreigners to re-emigrate to their respective home countries, the situation is not likely to change (Körner and Mehrländer 1986: 15–63). *Gastarbeiter* today are not temporary migrant workers but immigrant populations (Heckmann 1983).

The concept of ethnic minorities is rather vague and embraces a broad semantic scope because it does not refer to a homogeneous group but to a diversity of minorities which differ by religion, race, language, political affiliation, nationality and culture both from each other as well as from the majority group. The countries of origin of these minorities, their cultural and racial backgrounds, their legal status of residence as well as their nationality, motives for migration, the history of relationships between their home country and the host country, the length of their stay and their plans in terms of limited or permanent residence in the respective countries, all vary significantly throughout Europe. Nevertheless, certain features of social life, the generally negative way they are perceived by the host community, as well as their treatment within the criminal justice system seem to display rather important similarities. Although the status of a West Indian or a Moluccan or Surinamer coming to England or to the Netherlands for permanent settlement is clearly different from that of Turkish, Portuguese or Moroccan migrant workers in the FRG, France, Austria or the Netherlands, who in turn are different from various other groups of refugees, it seems clear that despite those differences in motives for migration and legal status of residence as well as citizenship, treatment by the majority group remains remarkably consistent. This is evident in various European countries where there are various ethnic minority groups with different legal status regarding residence, including minorities which have adopted the citizenship of the host countries. Prejudices against Turkish migrant workers in the FRG are much the same as those facing minorities recently arrived from the USSR or Poland. Both Moroccans and Moluccans face the very same problem of being marginalised in the Netherlands; Arabs with French nationality receive the same treatment as do other Arabs or Blacks from African countries in France.

The rather skewed distribution of research on the relationship between ethnic minorities, crime and criminal justice might be seen as reflecting powerful societal belief patterns, deeply rooted in an ever-present reservoir of xenophobia, ethno-centrism and general prejudice encouraged and activated in lower socio-economic groups through economic crises. These belief patterns with respect to crime involvement and crime causation are not unique. We may find such beliefs also, for example, with respect to the alcohol–crime link or the unemployment–crime link. But research in the field of minorities and crime is rather difficult due to the sensitivity of the topic and due to politicisation of the issue which is driven by organised interests on both sides. It follows that there is a danger that research also is polarised and restricted either to the study, description and explanation of disproportional crime involvement by minorities or to the study of discriminatory decision-making within the criminal justice system and maltreatment of minorities by its agents. The questions which are put forward and the answers which are sought, easily become controversial political issues; such politicisation is facilitated by the history of the treatment of minorities in Europe which shows how minorities have been preyed upon throughout the centuries.

In spite of the historical and cultural characteristics of each country's development and the variable status of minorities it does seem evident that there is a general focus on the crime proneness of ethnic minority groups. This is true also for criminological research which has centred on and is still preoccupied with the question of whether ethnic minorities actually commit more crime than the majority group. Although few studies have dealt with the problem of victimisation of minorities (Pitsela 1986; see also Mayhew *et al.* 1989: 43) there is considerable evidence that minorities are disproportionately affected by victimising events both in terms of criminal victimisation and in terms of other types of victimisation, for example work-place accidents, economic exploitation and trafficking in women from Third World countries for prostitution. Rather less research interest has focused on the relationship between ethnic minorities on the one hand and police and justice agencies on the other hand. Almost completely lacking is evaluative research dealing with the development and assessment of policies aimed at the reduction of discrimination and biased treatment in the different sectors of the justice system.

CRIME INVOLVEMENT OF ETHNIC MINORITIES

Superficial evaluation of police records on offences and offenders confirms that some minorities are disproportionally involved in crime commission when data are examined along ethnic variables.

However, some minorities do show up with under-average offender rates, for example Chinese and Asians in England and Wales or in the Netherlands and Spanish and Portuguese in the Federal Republic of Germany (Landeskriminalamt Nordrhein-Westfalien 1987), while others, such as black people, appear to commit offences above the average offender rate (Wiles 1989; Junger-Tas 1985). It seems obvious therefore that ethnic or minority variables do not have a uniform and consistent effect on crime rates (whether used as indicators of actual crime involvement or as an indicator of law-enforcement activities). Furthermore comparative analysis of regions and geographical units shows that rather considerable differences can be observed between offender rates even within the same minority group (Mansel 1986). Research suggests also that there are differences in the degree of crime involvement between generations of immigrants with the second or third generations born or raised in the immigration country displaying considerably higher offender rates than did the first generation of immigrants (Villmow 1983: 127–32). A tentative explanation could be that first-generation immigrants do experience (at least if they come from poor countries) an initial relative improvement of living conditions, housing, medical care, and so on, which counterbalances the differences between minority and majority groups, while second and third generations are more likely to become conscious of deprivation and socio-economic inequality as well as being subject to the conflict between the expectations of parents, families and relatives who are still strictly bound to traditional values of the ethnic group in question on the one hand and the values of the host country on the other, this conflict leading to intra-family conflicts and weakening of family controls (Bielefeld *et al.* 1982: 18–52; Aronowitz 1989: 280–4; Kaiser 1988: 599).

When looking at crime and offender data which are available for various European countries, we might come to the conclusion that on the whole most countries do indeed experience crime problems caused by ethnic minorities. We find in many European countries offender rates among certain groups of minorities which are two to four times as high as rates observed in society at large (Karger and Sutterer 1988; *Bericht der Bundesregierung* 1987; Andersson 1984; Craen 1984; Junger-Tas 1985; Walter 1987; Junger 1989). Even more impressive are the numbers of foreigners – within the prison population in some west European countries –

numbers which generally far exceed the respective proportions of ethnic minorities in the societies at large (see Figure 7.1). Although as can be expected, most of the crimes committed by minorities are property crimes, disproportional crime involvement as measured by police records is especially marked in the case of the most serious crimes such as violent crimes, sexual assaults, rape and robbery (Albrecht 1988a).

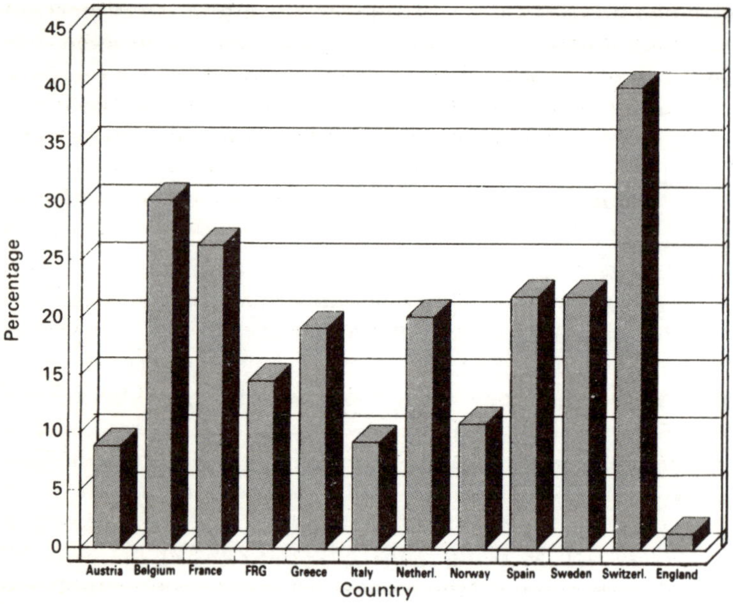

Source : Council of Europe 1988b

Figure 7.1 Foreign sub-populations in European prison systems, 1987

The basic questions arising out of these observations include the following:

1 Do police data show disproportionate crime involvement or disproportionate crime control?
2 Are minorities over-arrested relative to the number of criminal acts they commit or are they treated the same as the majority?
3 Finally, are police crime data merely over-estimating crime involvement of minorities through not accounting for relevant demographic or other variables?

Answers to these questions are not easily found. As research on crime and delinquency reveals, police data cover only a small proportion of those offences actually committed. Victimisation surveys found that only the minority of victimising events are reported to the police. It follows that police crime data could easily be biased against minorities. The research strategy regularly used to overcome the deficiencies of official crime data from police or court information systems relies on self-report surveys on the one hand and on victimisation surveys on the other. Unfortunately victimisation surveys are not a very good measure of the crime involvement of minorities because most victims do not know about their offender, at least in the case of property crimes, vandalism, burglary, and so on. On the other hand most victimisation surveys and self-report studies carried out in European countries so far have not included ethnic minorities, mainly because of methodological reasons. On the one hand language problems sometimes preclude minorities from interview-based research and, on the other hand, random sampling regularly leads to group sizes which are too small to produce meaningful results. Survey and interview-based research with respect to ethnic minorities in general poses the very same problems we face in intercultural and international comparative research (Albrecht 1989a).

Very recently, an in-depth and comprehensive study on crime involvement among ethnic minority and majority juveniles has been carried out in the Netherlands (Junger 1989). This piece of research relies on both self-report measures of delinquency and crime and official crime data and includes three minority groups (Moroccan, Surinam and Turkish juveniles) as well as a group of Dutch juveniles matched to the minority groups with respect to socio-economic status, and so on. First, the results obtained from this study lend support to the conclusion that self-report data should not be seen to be superior to official crime data. Obviously, validity of self-report measures is not the same for the various ethnic groups (Junger 1989: 154). While validity was rather high for Dutch boys and Surinamers, it was low for Moroccans and Turks. Differences in validity thus are rooted in culture or religion rather than in ethnicity and self-report studies therefore are not a better way to estimate whether differences in crime involvement actually exist. Furthermore, as self-reporting covers a range of relatively minor delinquent and criminal acts and official crime data cover more serious and repetitive criminal behaviour, it seems justified to rely on official crime data when attempting to control crime rates for relevant non-ethnic variables. When comparing the above-mentioned ethnic groups and a group of Dutch boys who were matched to these groups according to socio-economic background, it was found that the differences observable at large were reduced significantly, although differences did not vanish completely (Junger 1989). It should be added that differences were observed also within the three ethnic minority groups – an observation which is consistent with data from other countries pointing to varying degrees of crime involvement among ethnic minorities.

In the FRG similar research results could be obtained when comparing groups of German and Turkish juveniles with similar socio-economic backgrounds. The latest government security report for Austria dealt with a comparative analysis of crime involvement of both *Gastarbeiter* and other minority groups and of the host Austrian population. It is concluded that the *Gastarbeiter* commit considerably fewer serious offences than the (comparable) majority group (*Bericht der Bundesregierung* 1987: 86). In a small-scale study carried out in the south of the FRG it could be shown that putting the focus on the number of offenders rather than on numbers of offences is too narrow and probably misleading. Besides the fact that no differences between the minority juveniles and young adults aged 14 to 21 and the corresponding group of German citizens could be found with respect to the annual offender rate, the study revealed that when taking into account the number of offences committed by each offender, ethnic minority juveniles were contributing considerably less to the annual offence load than did their German counterparts (Oppermann 1986). Furthermore, re-offending or recidivism does not seem to be more common among minorities (Steffen 1983). On the other hand, American research came up with results which suggest that once involved in crime, ethnic minorities commit crimes at the same rate as do majority offenders (although prevalence of offending is obviously higher in the minority group; Petersilia 1985).

Summarising the available evidence on crime commission among ethnic minorities we may conclude that, if proper controls are included in research designs, the sometimes enormous differences between certain ethnic minorities and national majorities appear to fade away.

VICTIMISATION AND ETHNIC MINORITIES

A rather well-known phenomenon concerns the overlapping of offender and victim roles. Criminological research has revealed that those individuals with the highest risk of violent offending are also those with the highest risk of becoming the victim of a violent crime (Hough and Mayhew 1983: 21). Homicide is the leading cause of death among young black males in metropolitan areas of the USA, while young black males are disproportionately represented in the population of violent offenders. The victimisation studies conducted so far in European countries (in England, the Netherlands and the FRG) have also found higher rates of victimisation for ethnic minorities (Jones *et al.* 1986; Mayhew *et al.* 1989: 50; Home Office 1981; Junger and von Hecke 1988; Arnold 1983). Although these differences in victimisation rates between ethnic minorities and majority groups may be reduced when controlling for other non-ethnic variables which can be assumed to determine the level of victimisation (risk such as the type of neighbourhood, demographic and socio-economic background or routine activities of victims, and so on), the effects of victimisation could be more severe at least for certain sub-groups among ethnic minorities. When considering intra-family violence, for example, vulnerability of minority women and children is likely to be reinforced by their weak legal position as foreigners which may be made even worse by permanent separation or divorce. Furthermore, knowledge about available services is not widespread among these groups; the traditional subordinate positions of women in certain ethnic minority groups and language problems may add to the extent of victimisation (Hagemann-White 1981).

Non-criminal victimisation has to be taken into account too. Abortion rates (which perhaps indicate certain social problems) among ethnic minority women in the FRG are far higher than rates among the host German population (Bärtling *et al.* 1982). Estimates in the FRG indicate that accident rates among migrant workers are twice those among German workers. Additionally migrant workers are more at risk from exploitative employment conditions, with employers hiring immigrants on a non-contractual basis which allows avoidance of social security payments and other social benefits.

IS THERE DISCRIMINATION AGAINST ETHNIC MINORITIES IN THE SYSTEM?

The nature and sources of discrimination

The police, public prosecutors and courts are sometimes charged with discriminating against ethnic minorities. But as, virtually everywhere, up to 95 per cent of all crimes recorded by police are reported by the public and detection of a relatively small proportion of crimes is due to the activities of police themselves, and furthermore, as a correspondingly small number of offences are cleared up by police investigations, which are independent from evidence and information made available by the victim or the witness, it seems clear that research efforts designed to analyse selective and biased law enforcement should concentrate on reporting behaviour first. The victim of crime is the gatekeeper of the criminal justice system, apart from some fields of law enforcement such as with drugs, where traditional reactive police strategies have been replaced by proactive and aggressive styles of policing. But research on reporting behaviour and the role ethnic variables play is rather scarce and as far as criminological surveys on victims or witnesses of crime have covered variables such as perceptions of the nationality or race of the offender, research results are far from unambiguous. On the one hand, minority victims of crime seem to be slightly more reluctant to report an offence if the offender has the same national or ethnic background (Pitsela 1986: 340). This supports the assumption of under-reporting of ethnic minority crimes – especially if one takes into account the fact that a substantial proportion of personal crimes committed by ethnic minorities are committed within the minority group (Stevens and Willis 1979: 38; Sessar 1981). On the other hand, ethnic minority offenders seem to run a somewhat higher risk of being reported when analysing general reporting behaviour on the basis of victimisation surveys (Pease 1984; but see also Killias 1988, who found no association between ethnicity and reporting risk in Switzerland). Additionally it should be noted that research evidence suggests that ethnic minorities are disproportionately represented in the field of small, petty offences such as shoplifting. Ethnic minority offenders face a somewhat higher risk to be reported to the police when committing shoplifting or offences at the place of work (Blankenburg 1973; Kaiser and Metzger-Pregizer 1976).

But although there might be some effect of over-reporting on ethnic minorities, basically the victim's decision to report a crime is dependent upon his or her assessment of the seriousness of the offence – not upon the characteristics of the offender.

As far as discrimination within the criminal justice system is concerned, two dimensions should be identified:

1 a subjective dimension including attitudes, perceptions, verbal behaviour of police and criminal justice staff;
2 an objective dimension referring to decision-making, e.g. decision outcomes in terms of arrests, dismissal of cases, charging offenders, adjudication, sentencing, prison regimes and parole.

With respect to attitudes and perceptions there is some evidence that racist attitudes are present in police forces (Junger 1989; *Minderheden Bulletin* 1984; Carr-Hill 1987). Basically we may assume that those employed in the criminal justice system, including the police, do not differ very much from the public in terms of attitudes and perceptions, so it is reasonable to expect a corresponding structure of prejudices. However, as we know from research on the relationships between attitudes and behaviour, attitudes are in general not very good predictors of actual behaviour.

Turning to the field of decision-making and behaviour within police and criminal justice, we find that data do not indicate biases in making arrests although complaints about police harassment of minority juveniles are quite often heard in France, England, the Netherlands and in the FRG, where the police are criticised for giving black people too much negative attention (Bielefeld *et al.* 1982; Humphrey 1972; Carr-Hill 1987; D.J. Smith and Gray 1983; Junger 1989). Participant observation in the Netherlands revealed that black people were among those who attracted disproportionate attention from the police in terms of stop and search procedures (although this did not result in a higher arrest rate: Junger-Tas 1984a: 64). But, as is the case with respect to the analysis of criminal involvement of minorities, it is important to analyse the extent of use of stop and search procedures and of other police interventions both for minority and majority groups, from the same socio-economic background. Research on this issue has come up with rather divergent results. While it has been argued that in England, Blacks are stopped by police more often than Whites and that a higher proportion of encounters between minorities and police were of an adversarial nature (which might explain the apparently higher figure of formal complaints against police among ethnic minorities: Stevens and Willis 1981), Dutch research has pointed to the fact that, at least with respect to stopping vehicles, a higher rate of driving without a valid licence among ethnic minorities (With 1984) may account for differential patterns of suspicion. In a small-scale study in the FRG on attitudes of German, Turkish and Italian male juveniles toward police behaviour, and on the juveniles' evaluation of their encounters with police, it was found that German juveniles (who were matched to minority juveniles on the basis of socio-economic status), felt more strongly than did their Turkish and Italian counterparts that the streets and areas they lived in were controlled intensively by the police. Furthermore, a somewhat larger proportion of German boys complained about police behaviour and stressed the rudeness of the police. A relatively small proportion of Turkish juveniles complained about police behaviour, these complaints being based on the view that police discriminated against Turkish juveniles (Staudt 1983). According to this study, differences occurred in terms of attributing different motives to police activities (probably sometimes backed up by racist or discriminating verbal behaviour) and not in terms of differential strategies adopted by police in controlling minority and other youth. Similar results are available from England, where it was shown that more West Indians than Whites produced generalised complaints against police although the proportions of complainants referring to specific incidents did not differ (Tuck and Southgate 1981: 34–41).

It is interesting that minorities appear to be less tolerant about crime and criminals; this was demonstrated by a recent study on attitudes towards crime and criminal justice agencies. In the population surveyed, evidence was found among minorities for a stronger commitment to harsh penalties (including the death penalty) as well as to deterrence as a primary aim of sentencing and corrections. We may add that a substantial proportion of this minority group felt that the courts were restricting police too much in their efforts to control criminals and investigate crime (Pitsela 1986). But as far as perceptions of the performance of the criminal justice system are concerned, clear differences exist between various ethnic groups. While, for example, in the FRG, Greeks do not differ from the German population in their evaluation of the police and courts, black people in the UK lack confidence in the criminal justice system as well as being less satisfied with the performance of police after a crime is reported (Brown 1984; Mayhew *et al.* 1989: 28–9).

Making arrests and charging suspects

With respect to police decision-making on arrest, a consensus seems to exist among criminologists: the probability of being arrested assuming that the same number and type of offences have been committed, is more or less the same for minority and majority group offenders. We may add that the probability of being arrested is extremely low in the case of most offences anyway (Petersilia 1985) and that police decisions about making arrests seem to be guided by characteristics of the offence (especially seriousness) in the first place. It should be emphasised again that the structure of police routine activities and deployment of police resources do not leave much room for discriminatory decision-making to influence entry to the criminal justice system – police respond to calls from the public who consequently have a significant influence on who becomes involved in the criminal justice process in the first place.

When looking at subsequent stages in the process we find contradictory research results. While it has been argued that in England minority juveniles are less often cautioned by police and are more often sent to court than are white juveniles (Crow 1987), data from the Netherlands and the FRG do not lend support to the assumption of there being a greater risk of minority suspects being charged (Albrecht 1987a; Junger-Tas 1981; Junger 1989). The main criteria in these countries upon which the decision to prosecute is based are prior record, offence seriousness and admission of guilt. On the contrary, there is some evidence that minority offenders are less often brought to court in the FRG and in England, probably indicating a larger proportion of petty offences or a larger proportion of cases with weak evidence (Walker 1988; Mansel 1989: 285; see also the complete summary of research in Villmow 1989). This is true even in the case of the very sensitive crime of rape where a recently published report on processing rape cases through the system revealed that foreigners suspected of having committed a rape are less often brought to court than are German suspects and furthermore that differential treatment of within-group rape (where offender and victim are from the same group) and rapes involving a German victim and a minority offender did not occur (Steinhilper 1986). Similar results are reported from Sweden (Andersson 1984).

With respect to offenders of foreign nationality, a higher risk of being held in pre-trial detention has been observed in the FRG and in Austria (Jehle 1985; Pfeiffer 1988; Hanak *et al.* 1984). It may be that foreign minority group offenders are considered to be bad risks because of the likelihood of their returning to their home country before the trial takes place. Furthermore, French research suggests that time spent in police lock-ups and in pre-trial detention seems to be extended in the case of minority offenders (Malewska-Peyre 1982; Carr-Hill 1987).

Research from the USA does support these findings which in general lead to the conclusion that the input to the criminal justice system seems to reflect fairly impartial decision-making. Petersilia (1985) found, in a comprehensive study on racial disparities in the justice system, that at the front end of the process the system seems to treat white offenders even more severely and minority offenders more leniently.

Sentencing

There is evidence that discrimination has only a minor influence on sentencing. In countries where research on this issue has been carried out, minority defendants are somewhat more likely to receive prison or custodial sentences and less likely to receive suspended sentences or probation (Junger 1989; Crow 1987; Petersilia 1985; Steinhilper 1986; Walker 1988). Of all the variables which have an influence on disposal, ethnic and minority status appears to add only very modestly to the variation in sentencing (see e.g. Walker 1988); the probability of receiving a custodial sentence is 12 per cent for white people, 14 per cent for Asians and 16 per cent for black people – if indeed it actually contributes to the explanation of disparity in sentencing at all (Albrecht 1988b; Greger 1987). In the case of less serious crimes it can be suggested that equity in sentencing is present and is due to the extensive use of simplified procedures and the development of bureaucratic and administrative routines in sentencing as a response to a large volume of cases (see Albrecht 1987b for a summary of research). As ethnicity is a diffuse status variable, its impact on sentencing should be less pronounced or even non-existent where a consistent set of offence and offender-related characteristics (seriousness of the offence, prior record) points to rather obvious sentencing strategies. According to this assumption it is only an inconsistent set of characteristics which triggers the effects of what would otherwise be seen as the impact of ethnicity. Research seems to support this proposition (Unnever and Hembroff 1988) although the range of cases where ethnicity may become a powerful criterion in sentencing are rather few.

It has been assumed also that the relatively minor effects of ethnic variables on sentencing outcomes might be due to the fact that many serious personal crimes committed by minority offenders, involve a minority victim, and that the influence of ethnicity on sentencing might be greater for crimes committed by minority offenders against victims from the majority group. Research from the USA underlines the importance of analysing these groups separately. Although research in Europe on this topic is scarce, what there is does not (as has been mentioned above) strongly support the presence of this type of discrimination.

Social services within the criminal justice system and ethnic minorities

As most criminal justice systems have provision for social enquiry reports by probation departments or other officials of the court, the question arises as to how those report providers are performing in the case of minority offenders. Besides rather general observations indicating that serious problems in handling ethnic minority offenders within probation departments and similar agencies do exist, assessment is difficult because research dealing with this aspect of the criminal justice process is still lacking. Qualitative research from England demonstrates the existence of race bias in social enquiry reports both in a negative and a positive way (Waters 1988). But nevertheless when considering the importance of probation and other social services for the criminal justice system, further research is urgently needed to uncover the role and relevance of ethnicity in social inquiry reports, and its relationship to sentencing recommendations for both custodial and non-custodial disposals.

What happens after sentencing: administrative decisions and prison regimes

As an ethnic minority offender who does not have citizenship or right of residence may be expelled and deported to his or her home country once convicted and sentenced, decision-making processes within those administrative bodies which implement the relevant laws is of paramount importance. As statutes regulating deportation and expulsion as for example in the FRG, grant large discretionary power (Hailbronner 1984), it is not surprising that research demonstrated large variation both in the criteria adopted in decision-making and in decision outcomes (Albrecht and Pfeiffer 1979). Research concerning the role of these administrative bodies in responding to criminal or deviant behaviour of foreigners in general is sadly lacking and, unfortunately, details of the prison regime have not attracted much attention either.

The way a prison sentence is served varies considerably from one country to another. Recently collected data on the prison system in the FRG revealed that ethnic minorities who do not have German nationality are in fact experiencing a different kind of prison regime from German inmates. The data very clearly show that foreign prisoners are participating disproportionately less in furlough and home leave programmes. Furthermore, certain groups of inmates coming from South America and African or Arab countries can experience extreme isolation as these prisoners cannot maintain contact with the corresponding minority group outside prison (Albrecht 1989b). Whether treaties on the transfer of sentenced offenders and statutes on judicial aid will contribute to the alleviation of these problems is not yet clear. There is, however, some evidence that only a small number of foreign prison inmates would apply for being transferred to their home countries.

SUMMARY AND CONCLUSIONS

1 The research on crime involvement of ethnic minorities which is available for European countries indicates that if proper controls are introduced in research designs, crime is not more widespread among ethnic minorities than among comparable majority groups.

2 Ethnic minorities do not cause exceptional crime problems; crime among ethnic minorities reflects marginalisation and structural problems in societies.
3 Basically, explanations of crime among ethnic minorities should rely on the same set of variables which is used in explaining crime in general. Evidence does not exist to suggest that ethnic variables might be useful and meaningful in etiological research. Rather, it would be worth while to carry out research on the question of why majorities in societies are so interested in the crime proneness issue and why belief patterns which associate aliens and ethnic minorities with danger are so powerful.
4 Research on victimisation among ethnic minorities should be extended. Obviously victimisation rates are higher in these groups and effects of victimisation might be reinforced by marginal positions which hinder adequate access to relevant institutions.
5 Research on ethnic minorities and criminal justice is rather limited and in general piecemeal. Despite the dangers which might be inherent in a system of monitoring of ethnic and alien minorities within the criminal justice system, systematic and continuing data collection is needed in order to identify those points in the process where minority-related problems occur.
6 Research carried out up to now reveals that there is less evidence for discriminatory treatment at the front end of the process while differential treatment can be observed in prison regimes.
7 Discriminatory treatment occurs in terms of the use of offensive verbal or other harassing behaviour (e.g. stop and search) which may not affect the actual outcome of the process but nevertheless may be destructive for the relationship between minorities and justice agencies.
8 Although it seems promising to promote better relations between minorities and police and justice agencies by training staff, it should be noted that neither police nor other criminal justice personnel can be made accountable for the problems with race relations or relations between ethnic groups in general. Therefore training of professionals in criminal justice alone cannot be seen to represent the ultimate cure for these problems.
9 For a substantial portion of ethnic minorities in European

countries encounters with the criminal justice system include the risk of expulsion and deportation. It should be accepted that this type of reaction should be used only in cases of most serious crimes or persistent offending.

10 Basic remedies for problems of ethnic minorities and criminal justice can be derived from the theories outlined earlier. Whatever else may be undertaken, opportunities to overcome deprivation and to develop bonds to conventional society should be increased. As most of our societies appear not to be capable of achieving this for the traditional marginal groups, the numbers of which seem to have grown considerably in recent years, we should perhaps not be too optimistic.

© 1991 Hans-Jörg Albrecht

Part three

Policies and Problems

Chapter eight

Police co-operation within western Europe

Cyrille Fijnaut

INTRODUCTION

The political discussion on the subject of the unification of the Internal Market within the EC by the end of 1992, and in particular the debate on the elimination of border controls of individual citizens at the national frontiers of the member states, has turned the subject of international police co-operation into 'hot news' virtually overnight. Reinforcement and re-structuring of mutual co-operation between the police agencies of the countries involved is being urged all round, both with a view to the enforcement of one common immigration policy and to the maintenance of law and order, in particular the fight against serious crime including terrorism.

In order to avoid disappointment arising from unrealistically high expectations of the progress which could be made in police co-operation, I shall not just review the degree of progress which has actually been achieved to date but shall also examine the obstacles which stand in the way of its further advancement. Rather, I shall present a review of the several stages which police co-operation in western Europe has passed through during recent decades and shall consider the problems which have been associated with it.

Also I shall illustrate the extent to which the 'economic' unification of Europe has enhanced and even multiplied the problem of co-operation by referring to the experience of the Benelux countries (Belgium, Netherlands and Luxembourg) and by considering the impact of the Accord, regarding the elimination of controls at the common frontiers by 1990, which was signed on 14 June 1985 at Schengen between the Benelux countries, the Federal Republic of Germany (FRG) and France.

A FLASHBACK TO THE PAST

The police forces of western Europe have been working together for some time. Indeed how could they not work together given the number of countries contained within this relatively small area? However, it was not until the beginning of the nineteenth century that this co-operation really began to materialise. The best known example is from the mid-nineteenth century when the police of the German states co-operated in their fight against the political opposition to their own authority (Siemann 1985).

It was in 1898, at a secret conference in Rome, that police co-operation really started to spread across Europe. This was prompted by a determination to confront the violent anarchism of the time. All previous attempts towards the formation of a combined form of co-operation between the police agencies of western European countries having failed, Interpol was founded at long last in 1923. The background was of a political nature again. The aim was to create a means by which to maintain order and security in the continent of Europe which had become turbulent and politically unstable after the First World War.

Some forty years later, after the Second World War, there was not a similarly far-reaching initiative. At that time only Interpol was reinstated (Fijnaut 1987). However, one should not lose sight of the fact that under the stress of the Cold War beside this more or less overt form of police co-operation, real co-operation between the (new!) intelligence services in western Europe and the USA was established to contain communist zealots (Barnes 1981, 1982). Perhaps this development prevented international police co-operation being remoulded in a radical way.

The successive forms of police co-operation were all mainly aimed at improving the exchange of intelligence. However, one of the side-effects was a degree of harmonisation of operational practice method and equipment, particularly in the area of crime investigation. During the 1950s this was extended with formal judicial co-operation, in the form of 'small judicial aid'. However, this was actually also one of the achievements resulting from the conclusion of the 'European Treaty on the International Judicial Aid in Criminal Cases' in 1959. International judicial aid can be defined as the assisting of one country's penal process by another on the basis of mutual treaties.

From Interpol to TREVI

Compared with the rather slow evolution of internationalisation of criminal investigation up until the 1960s, its development ever since can safely be described as turbulent. It does not lend itself to easy analysis. The thread I shall follow is that the leading role which could have been played by Interpol has in fact been taken over by TREVI, the consultative body of the European Community dealing with matters of internal security.

Undoubtedly Interpol had, even during the 1970s, rendered great service to the police of western Europe and North America as far as the exchange of information about goods, people and criminal cases were concerned (Ferand and Schlanitz 1975; Nepote 1970). But this did not stop Interpol being sharply criticised especially in German, British and Dutch police circles. Although it was adequately equipped to investigate crime (including ever-expanding organised crime), according to the critics, Interpol had seriously failed to make a tactical and strategic analysis of the development of the pattern of crime with which it was dealing. The congress of the *Bund Deutscher Kriminalbeamter* (Association of German CID officers), which took place in Wiesbaden in 1974 was the first occasion on which this criticism had been expressed in plain and unequivocal terms.

Similar criticisms have followed since then by various influential authors, although they have each proposed to solve the problem in different ways. Some of them, like Horst Herold, who was the head of the *Bundeskriminalamt* (Federal Criminal Police Office) at the time, felt that Interpol would have to be altered, on the one hand through extensive modernisation of the information and documentation side of its operation and on the other by forming teams of experts who would assist with major investigation operations in the various countries.

But aside from that, Herold argued, there certainly was a task for the European Community (EC). It would have to facilitate mutual international judicial aid (see above) which he considered to be too much judicial and insufficiently police-oriented. That way the internationalisation, that is the standardisation of the widely diverging police systems, would be stimulated and criminal law would eventually become harmonised within the member states. According to Herold, the EC would at one and the same time have to see to it that the police judicial aid in the form of 'small frontier traffic' would be generally practised in the borderland between the affiliated states (Herold 1974).

Others, on the contrary, left Interpol out of the reckoning altogether. While they did not propose that the 'Parisian letterbox' be merely done away with, they did defend the 'Europol' idea within the EC. In the philosophy of Rolf Grunert, the Head of the *Bund Deutscher Kriminalbeamter*, this meant that the EC would not only have to harmonise criminal law and to simplify international aid, but also have to create a supranational criminal investigation department which would play an important part in the co-ordination of international investigations and would, in the case of some crimes, that is to say internationally organised crimes and serious contraventions of EC regulations, be able to launch investigations in its own right. Subsequently this new department would, he proposed, also be responsible for technical support of criminal investigation (for example in fields of dactyloscopy, photography, voice analysis and laser technology) and for the training of detectives (Gruner 1974).

Moreover there were in those days people like Jan Blaauw, who preferred the middle course (Blaauw 1974). He argued for the formation of a European Central Office within Interpol, for regular international and regional consultation between the chiefs of criminal investigation departments in Europe, for the setting up of international detective teams as appropriate for joint investigations in a European context and for the development of general facilities for international criminal investigation in Europe such as radio communications systems for the benefit of observation teams. On top of this he was in favour of simplifying mutual judicial aid and of harmonising legislation within the EC.

The reaction of Interpol, which at the time consisted mainly of French policemen, was one of some rigidity; they indicated that they would prefer to leave things as they were. They rejected the regionalisation of Interpol through the formation of an organisation like the proposed 'Europol' arguing that it would be unworkable because a number of criminal organisations operated both inside and outside Europe. They refused to give any emphasis to the executive aspects of task performance because this was said to be in conflict with the sovereignty of the affiliated states; if that were to be the case, foreign police officers would actively be involved in the application of national criminal law, which would be seen as unacceptable. They also rejected the idea of setting up regional conferences which, they argued, would not be viable without the resources of the central services in the different countries (Langlais 1974).

Progress was made, however, as far as attempts to combat drug abuse were concerned. It was probably no coincidence that this happened at the same time as the initiative taken in 1971 by President Pompidou of France to co-ordinate western European efforts to fight the traffic and consumption of illegal narcotic drugs. Interpol appointed several liaison officers at the organisation's general office in Saint Cloud (which is near Paris), each of whom had responsibility for co-ordinating investigations in given parts of western Europe. Seven years later a small unit was added which was responsible for making tactical and strategic analyses of the narcotics traffic throughout the whole of western Europe (Littas 1979). This concession did little to satisfy the critics of the 1970s. The FRG police in particular were still attracted by the idea of a 'Europol', although some influential individuals like Horst Herold stuck to their original views as described above (Krusell 1980; Herold 1980; Jeschke 1980). Nor did the criticism of those who were opposed to Interpol die down either. One of the leading criminal investigation chiefs of the Metropolitan Police, J. Huins, while lecturing at the Police Staff College at Bramshill, recited a long list of defects and drawbacks with Interpol before putting the question

> What good is the membership of Interpol, if Interpol doesn't adequately respond to the executive needs of the European police; if Interpol won't hear of regionalisation, not even of training, in and outside Europe; if Interpol won't . . . ?
>
> (Huins 1980)

In spite of criticism continuing up to the present day, the staff of Interpol have nevertheless maintained their view of the organisation as a world-wide police intelligence service (Brugger 1981).

Things progressed during the 1970s. Both formal and informal consultative and co-operative bodies which have relevance to police investigation, have been created throughout Europe. The Cross Channel Conference and the European Capital Chiefs of Police Conference are two examples (Fijnaut and Visser 1985). In

1978 there was an agreement between Germany and France about their common border and since 1969 there had been a number of less formal arrangements in the border area near Aachen within the framework of 'NEBEDEACPOL' the *Niederlandisch-Belgisch-Deutschen-Polizeikonferenz* (the Dutch-Belgian-German Police Conference) (Seifried 1981). The *Arbeitsgruppen zur Bekämpfung der Rauschgiftkriminalität* (the Working Groups for the Fight Against Drug Crime) which was set up in the mid-1970s at the initiative of the German police in co-operation with neighbouring authorities is also important (Salewsky 1974). Furthermore, we should not forget that ever since the 1960s European police services have been co-operating, largely without the knowledge of Interpol, with the major federal police services in North America, particularly with the Federal Bureau of Investigation (FBI), the Drugs Enforcement Administration (DEA) and the Royal Canadian Mounted Police (Barnes 1981, 1982; Fijnaut 1983) in the sphere of political intelligence work and more traditional organised crime including illicit traffic in narcotics.

These and other new consultative bodies have furthered the development of international co-operation in respect of both the dissemination of information and of operational activity, such as the exchange of communications machinery (such as walkie-talkies) and procedural agreements concerning operations on each other's territory. But by far the most significant development in the field has been the creation and recently the enlargement of TREVI.

The initiative to set up this consultative body, which was institutionalised within the European Political Co-operation of the EC, was taken by the European Council in Rome in 1975. The Council then agreed that the respective Ministers of Internal Affairs would regularly get together to discuss issues of order and security. This decision became much more important a year later when on 29 June 1976 in Luxembourg, these ministers adopted a resolution to the effect that a number of study groups were to be established as part of a body which was to be called TREVI, a name derived from the famous fountains in Rome. TREVI was founded against the background of extensive violence committed by extremists in several European countries in 1975 and 1976; under the supervision of the European Council these groups were intended to stimulate co-operation in the fight against terrorism and would exchange information about the organisation, equipment and training of police units (Schoutheete 1980: 131–46).

The decision to create TREVI illustrates very well the impetus behind internationalisation; as soon as there was an attack on the establishment of the European countries in the form of terrorism, there was an incentive to establish police co-operation. It should be emphasised therefore that the founding of TREVI was an important move even at the very moment of its foundation – important because the co-operation between the police forces of western Europe was thereby raised to a level which surpassed anything which had been accomplished or even proposed during the previous hundred years. It was significant also because the co-operation brought about by the creation of TREVI extended political co-operation between the member states of the EC into the sphere of domestic politics, where it can in every respect rank with the co-ordinating bodies of the European Political Co-operation existing in the sphere of foreign politics. TREVI also acted as a springboard from which other initiatives, concerning information, operations and organisation, could be taken (Fijnaut 1982: 52–7).

The extent to which this potential has been exploited is hard to establish with certainty, largely because of the secrecy and confidentiality surrounding much of TREVI's activity. But it is clear that TREVI has borne fruit particularly in connection with terrorism and other forms of extremism. Until recently there were two TREVI study groups working in this field, one occupied with the exchange of intelligence about (potential) attacks and the (suspected) attackers and one studying mainly the operational aspects of action against terrorist and extremist groups.

Having originally narrowed its focus in this way, TREVI then quite dramatically changed the situation. On 21 June 1985 the TREVI Ministers (the Ministers for Home Affairs and Justice in their own countries) decided to form a third study group which was to study methods and techniques of fighting international crime such as armed robberies and traffic in narcotic drugs and weapons.

The precise reason for the broadening of TREVI's brief is not entirely clear. Was it because in some cases there (probably) has been a close relationship between terrorism – the way it has, more explicitly than before, been manifest in various shapes in recent years – and other forms of organised crime? Examples of this are the relationships between terrorist movements and Mafia groupings in Italy in the sphere of the weapon trade, and between the terrorist attacks of the IRA and its extortion and smuggling activities in the border area of Northern Ireland. Or perhaps it was due to the increasing tendency for instance within the European Council to look upon organised crime as an issue of European public order? Or, one might decide, perhaps somewhat facetiously, that western European politicians must continuously create new stimuli to keep alive the idea of the European Community.

Whatever may have been the reason for this decision, the fact remains that it may have far-reaching consequences for the operational and instrumental organisation of police investigation in western Europe, as long as, that is, it is put into effect energetically. In view of the resolution adopted by the European Council on 24 April 1986 in The Hague, this could indeed well be the case. The resolution adopted on that day contained the seeds out of which an independent 'Europol' could grow within the European Community. This 'prophecy' of increasing co-operation is all the more legitimate because at The Hague conference the TREVI Ministers also decided that the future activities of the study groups and the Committee of Higher Officials would have to be co-ordinated and evaluated by a permanent office, the so-called Troika, which would consist of the immediate past president of TREVI, the current president and his successor (Fijnaut 1986).

Evidently this reform of TREVI more or less implies a choice between the alternatives which had been brought forward in the discussion about Interpol during the 1970s. Since that choice was to Interpol's disadvantage, why had Interpol not worked harder to be more closely involved in this international development? The answer lies, I think, in the fact that Interpol is in the final analysis not much more than an international information centre and is not incorporated into international political structures and therefore cannot be a proper instrument for adequate management for as delicate an issue as terrorism.

Bear in mind also that the fight against terrorism was a most ticklish affair for Interpol in the mid-1970s because it had been sharply criticised in the USA and in some European countries for neglecting a clause contained in Article 3 of its own statutes, which prohibited interference with political, military, religious or racial matters – which is what its investigation into oppositional groups and religious groups was taken to be. In other words, explicit and full-scale participation in the fight against terrorism could have endangered the entire covenant of Interpol. Interpol subsequently gave in somewhat reluctantly, but by then it was too late to maintain or even restore the monopoly which it had previously held in western Europe (Garrison n.d.; Gulbinowcz 1978).

UNDISCUSSED ISSUES AND FORGOTTEN PROBLEMS

The foregoing overview of international police co-operation in western Europe clearly shows that its evolution during recent decades did not take place without its fair share of problems. Major differences of opinion surfaced concerning the shape which was to be given to this co-operation and these disagreements and occasional fierce debates have produced today's extremely complicated structure.

A degree of dissent amongst those who were trying to build co-operative structures was only part of the problem. While these problems were apparent to all, there were also a number of latent difficulties. There were indeed many subjects which were either not discussed at all or which were given very little attention but should be considered if we wish to make real progress towards co-operation in the near future.

First, there is the problem of terrorism and other forms of organised crime which are frequently used to argue in favour of further internationalisation. One of the biggest difficulties is the fact that there is only a poor understanding of the extent, nature and evolution of organised (political) crime in western Europe. We can assume, based on reasonably reliable sources, that during the past twenty years, certain kinds of terrorism and violent activism (this category including the activities of radical protest groups which use violence to achieve their ends) have increased, not only in larger countries such as the FRG, but also for example in Belgium (Bruggeman and Luypaers 1986: 570–81).

Nevertheless, a realistic picture of the total phenomenon of organised crime is altogether lacking (Fijnaut 1985: 5–42; Schmid 1983). Over the past twenty years, serious studies of the subject have been limited to particular facets, countries and periods of time (Sack and Steinert 1984). Of course, absence of quantitative information on this subject makes it extremely difficult to estimate the need for co-operative international investigation in western Europe. The volume of terrorism is only part of the story; one must also consider how much police time is necessary and justified in order to achieve a certain degree of control over the problem, particularly in relation to the police resources which are available to fight other forms of crime (Fijnaut *et al.* 1985).

Referring to the FRG's approach to terrorism, Heinrich Boge raised the question in 1986 as to whether there might not be other more effective means for countering terrorism other than the deployment of the police (Boge 1985: 587–92; Plenel 1986: 7–20). By the same token, it could also be suggested that large-scale development of internationally organised investigation might, in the long run, be counter-productive by encouraging the further internationalisation of crime itself (McIntosh 1975).

Second, there are many questions about the functioning of existing institutions and regulations which have a bearing on further internationalisation. Indeed, we can learn much from looking closely at attempts at co-operation which have already taken place. Recent experience on the road to the internationalisation of crime investigation has, to my knowledge, never before been properly evaluated. An evaluation of Interpol and judicial internationalisation and of the new and lesser known forms of co-operation could be most instructive. Examples of such co-operation include TREVI, the German–French agreement on co-operation which was concluded in 1978, the co-operation in the borderland of the FRG, Belgium and the Netherlands (NEBEDEACPOL) and the agreement signed on 18 July 1960 entitled *Abkommen über die dienstlichen Beziehungen zwischen Deutschen und Belgischen Polizeibehörden im Grenzgebiet* (Agreement on the official relations between the German and Belgian police authorities in the borderland). It is certainly a matter of some importance to find out how these forms of co-operation have been operating in practice if one is proposing either to expand them or to replace them by other more far-reaching forms of co-operation.

Third, there are problems of control of international co-operation. As Rigaux said in 1985 (as had many others before and after him such as Dubois 1978; Orie 1983; Wijngaart 1980), the judicial co-operation which exists in western Europe has been promoted mainly for the following reasons: first, to prevent suspects, whom all the states concerned would like to prosecute, from having a refuge on the territory of one of them, and second, to enhance the containment of crimes which are seen as menaces to the different states in themselves.

Without doubting the legitimacy of these aims, I agree with Rigaux and others who maintain that the protection of suspects has never been given much consideration without any justification for this circumstance. Therefore it is my belief that if police co-operation in western Europe is to move forward on the track which we have previously described, we can within the context of what in the international jargon is sometimes referred to as 'fair administration of justice' not be anxious enough to pay attention to the legal protection of suspects (Swart 1984).

This can be done first by clearly defining a suspect's rights in new treaties and by creating possibilities to fight violations in court; in the absence of an effective, adequate court at a European level this must be undertaken at national level. Second, the judicial control of investigations which involve the crossing of frontiers will have to be improved, not only through the installation of (international) control by the offices of counsel for the prosecution existing in the various countries, but also especially with respect to all non-judicial aspects of this kind, by tightening up supervision by the Departments of Justice; these Departments could make arrangements concerning the number, location, competence and equipment of units that may engage in cross-border operations. Third, the political control of the administration of investigations in western Europe should be strengthened, either by the national Parliaments or, in view of TREVI and Interpol, by the European Parliament.

The best proof of the validity of my suggestion that we are dealing with forgotten problems was delivered during 1986 by the European Parliament and by the Council of Europe. These two institutions had produced and debated reports on how to counter organised crime in (western) Europe. I refer on the one hand to the report by Sir Jack Stewart-Clark on how to handle the drugs problem in the EC (European Parliament Working Documents 1986–7) and on the other hand to the report by Piet Stoffelen on international crime in the EC countries (Council of Europe 1986). Neither of these two reports pays even the slightest attention to the problems which I have identified above: the extent and content of organised crime, the effectiveness of the existing forms of police co-operation and the lack of legal protection for suspects. Raising some of these 'forgotten problems' would certainly have been justified, given the reports' recommendations for the formation of a 'European Police Information Office' and for devising

> a European framework agreement, if possible laid down in a legal instrument, maintaining a set of principles, conditions, and rules for . . . a practical, executive police cooperation between the individual member states on a bilateral or multilateral basis as well as for the accommodation of legislation concerning [the admissibility of] police fighting tactics, especially the issue of 'controlled deliveries' and the adjudication of police powers with respect to the monitoring of financial transactions and the seizure of illegally obtained money.
>
> (Council of Europe 1986; European Parliament Working Documents 1986–7)

A striking detail in these two reports is that they both voice an explicit preference for reinforcement for the task of Interpol within western Europe rather than an extension of TREVI. This makes it clear that there is a huge difference of opinion between individual national governments on the one hand and the members of the European Parliament and the Council of Europe on the other concerning the basis on which police co-operation in western Europe might proceed.

THE ECONOMIC UNIFICATION OF WESTERN EUROPE IN 1992 AND THE FURTHER INTERNATIONALISATION OF POLICE CO-OPERATION

The plans of the EC

When in 1986 the time had come to slow down somewhat the pace of the progress of internationalisation of police co-operation in western Europe in order to consider carefully what might be the next step, representatives of the EC member states were attaching their signatures to the Single European Act on 17 and 18 February of the same year. Article 13 of this Act amends Article 8a of the original EEC Treaty and stipulates that before 31 December 1992 the Community will achieve an internal market: in other words, an area without the barriers of national frontiers within which free traffic of goods, people, services and capital is guaranteed.

In order to be able to realise the Single Market on schedule, it will be necessary, according to the European Commission's White Book (which contains a list of all the questions that should be solved before 1993), for various measures to be taken by the

Council of Ministers with respect to the border control of people crossing national frontiers within the EC. The practical steps which the Commission has in mind include the following:

1 the elimination of police checks on entry and departure from territories of the various member states;
2 harmonisation of the legislation on narcotic drugs and firearms;
3 harmonisation of the laws on the rights of political asylum and the legal status of refugees;
4 harmonisation of visa policies;
5 harmonisation of extradition legislation.

On the face of it this would seem to contradict the final chapter of the Single European Act, which stipulates that no part of the preceding regulations will impede the right of member states to take such measures as they may deem necessary in order to conduct border controls on immigrants from non-EC countries and to counter terrorism, criminality, drug-trafficking and illegal trade of objects of art and antiques. However, this stipulation in fact indicates a degree of ambiguity in so far as not only the member states themselves but also the Council of Ministers are authorised to devise a policy with respect to these issues.

By mid-1989 there had not been much to see at EC level, which would indicate that they are energetically pursuing a policy concerning border controls. This is not hard to understand. One has only to think of statements made by Mrs Thatcher to realise that the economic unification of Europe is still a controversial political issue. The official negotiations on the concrete implementation of this Single European Act have only recently started and it should certainly not be lost sight of that it is an extremely difficult task to bring about a common policy with respect of border controls. Just how difficult it actually is can best be illustrated by the Benelux experiment and with the negotiations that are currently being conducted on the implementation of the Schengen Accord.

The experience of the Benelux Treaty and the Schengen Accord

A discussion of the Benelux Treaty is particularly interesting in the context of this chapter because it concerns an economic union (which was formed in the period 1958–60 between Belgium, the

Netherlands and Luxembourg) in which the border controls were removed from the internal frontiers. This Treaty may be seen as a test case for the EC after 1992.

If we examine what achievements this economic union has prompted in the area of immigration policy and more specifically in the area of police co-operation with a view to maintenance of public order and security, we find that the 'test case' has produced a number of interesting results.

In the first place, it can be established that through the implementation of a number of resolutions, the enforcement of the immigration laws in the three countries was harmonised in a number of ways. However, each of the three countries retained its own individual immigration law and, just as important, in a number of areas the enforcement of these laws is not harmonised at all, neither in practice nor in law. Also, the Dutch authorities are not happy about the way Belgium is carrying out border checks on their behalf at the Belgian border with France; for years, they have been maintaining that these border checks are not being made thoroughly enough. To remedy this, they posted their own officials of the *Koninklijke Marechaussee* near the Dutch–Belgian border in 1976 in order to monitor the traffic of people who may be entering via France and Belgium. Consequently it is no exaggeration to conclude that the Benelux experiment, at least in this respect, has failed. If the parties would wish to undo this failure, they would probably have to establish a common border patrol service. However, establishment of such a common agency is practically impossible because of political, governmental and financial reasons. The Netherlands therefore has little choice other than to try to keep any problems as manageable as possible through frequent dialogue with the Belgian government, in particular the Belgian Minister of Justice, who is responsible for the application of the Aliens Act.

The co-operation between the police forces of the Benelux countries has not grown spectacularly, to say the least. As early as 1962, a number of measures were adopted to advance co-operation which were embodied in the Benelux Treaty on extradition and judicial aid in criminal cases. This Treaty provided police officers with the legal right to pursue suspects across the border into the territory of one of the other Benelux countries and even to arrest suspects within 10 kilometres radius of the border; this is the so-called 'hot pursuit' clause. The Treaty also laid down the rules for the presence of law-enforcement officers in criminal investigations which are being carried out at their own request in another country. However, these measures, and particularly the 'hot pursuit' clause, were not defined in more detail until 1976. Even then, the measures applied only to the Dutch and Belgian provinces of Limburg on either side of the border. It was only from then on that some actual co-operation began to develop in day-to-day operations of the police agencies of Belgium and the Netherlands in this part of the common border area. They co-operated in such activities as the synchronisation of contingency plans, jointly conducted border checks, exchange of information bulletins and 'wanted' notices as well as access to each other's communication equipment. Across the remaining and indeed largest part of the common border area, co-operation continued to be a matter of ceremonial exchanges only, such as mutual visits at official openings of police stations.

Just as much, however, may be learnt from considering those areas in which co-operation has not progressed as by considering areas where progress has been made. There is still for example no satisfactory procedure which lays down the rules for mutual co-operation in an emergency or major investigation operation, although the need for such regulation has been felt for decades. The conflicting organisational structures of the police agencies in Belgium illustrate the point clearly. Apart from the *Rijkswacht* (National Police), there is the *Gerechtelijke Politie* (Judicial Police) as well as (in the larger towns) the municipal police. They are all authorised to act independently without consultation with each other or indeed their opposite numbers in the Netherlands and Luxembourg.

No efforts have ever been undertaken in the Benelux countries which have been specifically aimed at the harmonisation of the police organisations involved. This does not mean of course that some degree of harmonisation has not actually been established in recent years in a number of areas as a result of the informal exchange of information and a sharing of operational methods, but apart from this incidental harmonisation, the police organisations in the countries involved have all been through their own separate evolutionary process.

Progress has also been slow with respect to the criminal law, such as Firearms Laws and Narcotic Drugs Legislation. Even in spite of all the agreements that were concluded with a view to harmonisation of these laws, it did not work out according to plan, at least not between the Netherlands and Belgium. The Benelux countries are still a long way from following one common policy in these areas; the discrepancies are still extremely large.

Against the background of these experiences with Benelux, it is of course not surprising that the talks on the implementation of the Schengen Accord concerning the removal of controls at common frontiers, although projected to become effective in 1990, so far have yielded only very poor results (Tweede Kamer 1986–7). Yet in 1985–6 when it was signed, expectations were high. The working party which had been set up to study the problems of 'Police and Security' had been given the task of developing proposals on how to accomplish harmonisation of the policy on narcotic drugs, firearms and ammunition, terrorism and illegal organisations on the one hand and to devise proposals aimed at improvement of the quality of international judicial aid, the exchange of police information and border controls on the other. In mid-1987 the word was that these proposals had to be ready at the beginning of 1988. However, at the time of writing, the whole negotiating process has stopped. The main reason is quite simple: political disagreements between the governments concerned about the (solution of the) different questions are too great.

It is not hard to imagine that there is a great deal of opposition in the Netherlands (as there is in the UK) to the idea of the introduction of an identity card and even to the idea of a system of mandatory identification such as already exists in the neighbouring countries which are the co-signatories to the Schengen Accord. Neither does it require a great deal of imagination to realise that enormous criticism would be generated in the Netherlands by any proposal to change the prevailing criminal law policy on the subject of soft drugs in order to adjust it to the prevailing legislation on the subject in the neighbouring countries of the Federal Republic of Germany, Belgium and France. These are just two of the many problems that the members of the working party considering police and security will have to find solutions for in the coming months.

CONCLUSION

The internationalisation of police co-operation has made progress mainly whenever the security of the social order was, or seemed to be, under threat. Obviously the quintessence of the modern state – its sovereignty – and following naturally from this its monopoly of violence normally does not encourage such internationalisation. If for pressing reasons of security it is considered necessary to co-operate internationally, that co-operation will be organised in secret or through informal channels. The fact that such co-operation once organised has turned out to run relatively smoothly is largely because it has been mainly restricted to the exchange of intelligence on individuals, goods and incidents. The modest harmonisation of legislation policy and organisational structures which there has been has nearly always been forced by circumstance rather than having been a carefully planned political choice.

In view of this first conclusion, our second one must be that the plans of the EC for 1992 are extremely ambitious. The fact is that in the absence of any imperative to maintain security, the EC not only is aiming at intensifying the existing level of co-operation but also wishes to accomplish harmonisation of government policies on a wide range of policing matters. Furthermore, there is no suitable platform to take on the dialogue that is essential for making progress with such efforts. Also, we cannot ignore the fact that there is not one exhaustive comparative study of the organisation and operation of the various police agencies to inform this dialogue. Nor is there a study of the enforcement of all sorts of criminal law and of the actual enforcement of border checks on people crossing national frontiers.

Based on the experience gained so far with the Benelux experiment and the Schengen Accord, it can safely be stated that the plans for the EC from 1992 are far too ambitious. The major political governmental and legal differences between the EC countries will neither be overcome easily nor within such a short span of time. Not only are these differences too large in themselves, but also both the active and passive opposition to their elimination is too substantial to be ignored.

I think we should be more realistic. I would suggest that we make sure that by 1992 every effort is made to have the issue of border controls at the external frontiers sorted out and to have the immigration laws of the countries concerned harmonised only so far as is necessary to remove primary border controls to the external frontiers. It would be advisable to have a detailed proposal for the elimination of controls ready by 1992 based on the existing co-operation agreements such as those between the FRG and France and between the FRG and Austria; this would be a draft proposal for co-operation on a Europe-wide basis. Finally, in my opinion, efforts should be made within the EC towards a programme of research on the subject of police and security, parallel with research programmes on technological and economic subjects such as that of ESPRIT. The results of this programme would first and foremost have to be utilised towards harmonisation of the organisational structure of the various police agencies, criminal legislation and the police procedures in day-to-day operation (Klink 1987: 183–9).

© 1991 Cyrille Fijnaut

Chapter nine

Social development and the prevention of crime in France

A challenge for local parties and central government

Marie-Pierre de Liège

INTRODUCTION

Crime rates in modern France have followed similar trends to those in other European nations, especially Britain and the Federal Republic of Germany. Recorded offences showed regular, if erratic increases, throughout the 1970s and early 1980s (Figure 9.1 and Table 9.1). Between 1972 and 1984 recorded crimes rose by 119 per cent. While parallel trends occurred elsewhere, in France these were accompanied by political developments which led to crime prevention becoming a major focus for social policies. In this chapter the background to, and history of, these changes are explored and the distinctive aspects of the French model of crime prevention highlighted. As Figure 9.1 and Table 9.1 show, overall crime rates have apparently fallen in France since 1985.

BACKGROUND

Crime rates grew fairly steadily in France during the 1970s and early 1980s. More specifically numbers of minor offences increased sharply as did crime in cities. Thefts from cars, for instance, taking 1972 as a base year, had grown threefold by 1980 and fivefold by 1982 (Table 9.2). Burglaries doubled over the same period (Table 9.3). More dramatically, robberies with a female victim quadrupled between 1972 and 1980 and had grown by 750 per cent by 1985 (Table 9.4). While officially recorded crime figures were expanding markedly during this period feelings of fear of crime grew even more quickly amongst the French public.

Two reasons for this phenomenon can be advanced, the first is political, the second has to do with the criminal justice system. Fear of crime became a political issue in France in the 1970s. Questions

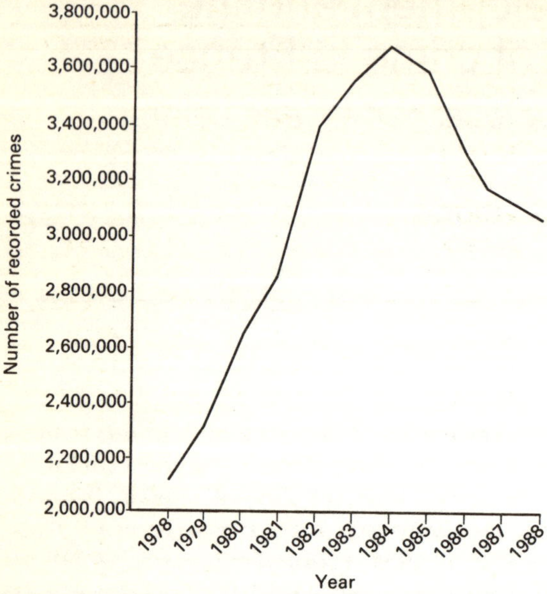

Source : Ministry of Justice 1989

Figure 9.1 Recorded crime in France, 1978–88

Table 9.1 Recorded offences in France, 1978–88

Year	*Total*	*% change*
1978	2,147,832	2.38
1979	2,330,566	8.51
1980	2,627,508	12.74
1981	2,890,020	9.99
1982	3,413,682	18.12
1983	3,563,975	4.40
1984	3,681,453	3.30
1985	3,579,194	-2.78
1986	3,292,189	-8.02
1987	3,170,970	-3.68
1988	3,132,694	-1.21

Table 9.2 Thefts from cars in France, 1972–88

Year	*Number*	*Index*	*% change*
1972	120,657	100	
1973	126,419	105	4.77
1974	165,594	137	30.98
1975	219,065	182	32.29
1976	240,570	199	9.81
1977	282,973	235	17.62
1978	300,160	249	6.07
1979	352,444	292	17.41
1980	431,840	358	22.52
1981	501,788	416	16.19
1982	627,944	520	25.14
1983	660,302	547	5.15
1984	720,360	597	9.09
1985	721,028	598	0.09
1986	652,448	541	– 9.51
1987	624,584	518	– 4.28
1988	675,032	559	1.09

Table 9.3 Burglaries in France, 1972–88

Year	*Number*	*Index*	*% change*
1972	20,791	100	
1973	22,989	111	10.57
1974	28,944	139	25.90
1975	32,858	158	13.52
1976	33,112	159	0.77
1977	36,113	174	9.06
1978	35,955	173	– 0.43
1979	39,850	192	10.83
1980	47,152	227	18.32
1981	51,501	248	9.22
1982	61,289	195	19.00
1983	70.593	340	15.18
1984	80,204	386	13.61
1985	79,751	384	– 0.56
1986	75,414	363	– 5.43
1987	73,696	354	– 2.28
1988	75,514	353	– 0.25

Table 9.4 Robberies with violence (female victim) in France, 1972–88

Year	*Number*	*Index*	*% change*
1972	3,678	100	
1973	4,319	117	17.42
1974	5,434	148	25.80
1975	7,294	198	34.22
1976	7,380	201	1.18
1977	8,736	239	18.37
1978	11,158	303	27.72
1979	13,346	363	19.60
1980	15,114	411	13.24
1981	18,106	492	19.79
1982	21,044	572	16.22
1983	23,893	650	13.53
1984	27,553	749	15.31
1985	28,079	763	1.90
1986	22,702	617	– 19.14
1987	21,580	587	– 4.94
1988	22,445	610	4.01

about rising crime were regularly raised in the battle between the parties of the right and those of the left. The mass media, especially the press, gave these stories full coverage, thus raising public awareness and levels of anxiety. At the same time, the economic crisis and the recession made many groups feel especially vulnerable.

Despite mounting public concern, the police and the courts, the conventional agencies of crime control, did not respond well. They were not geared to cope with minor crimes. Clear-up rates were usually only about 20–40 per cent. Heavy sentences, often custodial, followed conviction, but these were unsuccessful in effecting positive changes. Recidivism occurred in 50 per cent or more of cases where offenders were imprisoned.

CRIME PREVENTION POLICIES

As a result of the situation outlined above, two distinctive policy initiatives were pursued quite separately and without any apparent co-ordination. In the first of these the emphasis was on welfare policies, more specifically on social activities planned for young people. France already had an extensive commitment to preventive action directed through detached street workers. Some 6,000 of these worked on programmes organised and financed by the Ministry of Social Affairs.

In considerable contrast to this welfare approach, a policy of '*répression*' was being simultaneously pursued by the agencies of criminal justice. ('*Répression*' in France means strict enforcement of the criminal code by the police and the judiciary and the widespread use of imprisonment as a punishment.) A series of legislative changes between 1978 and 1981 reinforced this repressive approach.

THE NEW APPROACH

The recent history of crime prevention developments in France starts with the establishment of the Peyrefitte Commission in 1976. In response to apparent public concern with violent crime, a Commission was established to investigate violent crime and delinquency. The Commission was composed of a small elite group of high-profile individuals, who used the knowledge of experts to analyse the problems of crime in France and make recommendations for action. This Commission pointed to the problems of socio-economic disintegration, particularly in public housing areas in cities, as well as to the need for better building design. It also saw violence as a product of negative life experiences that might be tackled by treatment rather than punishment.

This Commission was chaired by M. Peyrefitte, who went on to become the Minister of Justice and so moved to implement the report by establishing a National Council on the Prevention of Violence (CNPD) and 'departmental' councils. Unfortunately, this National Council was not successful in stimulating many changes in local action, probably because its members were 'experts', not practitioners. Today its aims are

1 To develop a national policy on crime prevention: for that purpose the CNPD executive committee officials, composed of city administrations and of a large range of ministries, meet regularly to determine the general trends of their policy, prepares an annual report and sends each year an instruction to each departmental and municipal council giving recommendations for action. Gradually the ministries, which previously used to work on their own, learn to integrate the consequences of the new global approach in their policies. Inter-ministerial and

joint working groups are created each time a need appears (e.g. changing public attitudes, mediation, private enterprise involvement).

2 To organise and develop co-operation between local government, voluntary organisations and the private sector: the main idea for prevention of crime is that it is a challenge not only for professionals or experts but also for everyone, and that it must become a matter of lasting concern. It is also assumed that a significant number of local activists and of resources are in fact already targeted at the area. But very often these services ignore each other and then organise their action in an inappropriate way. In some areas one could find more than a hundred social workers intervening at the same time but separately, while in another district nothing at all was organised. The key aims of the national and local councils are partnership and co-operation. In most towns and cities the local team council now meets and works regularly together, to plan their action, to discuss their results and difficulties. However, if local government and voluntary organisations are now used to working together, the involvement of the private sector is still very patchy except, of course, for matters such as training and employment.

3 To fund prevention programmes: the CNPD through its budget funds two types of programmes. It funds crime prevention contracts with local authorities and special programmes, both new and original, run by those experienced in the field of crime prevention or prevention of recidivism and considered to be particularly interesting and exemplary.

4 To inform the public and train it in its civic responsibilities: several national and a large range of local information campaigns have been organised and financed by the CNPD (TV media, weeks for prevention, conferences . . .).

5 To examine the effectiveness of programmes undertaken: the lack of studies (research and evaluation) was very significant in France especially in these fields. The CNPD with its system of annual contracts is very helpful for promoting evaluation studies which can be carried out by local researchers as well as by local partners themselves (self-evaluation).

A left-wing government came into office in France in May 1981. During their years in opposition they had attacked both repressive policies and the exploitation of fear of crime for political purposes.

They were immediately faced with two problems. One was a 'crime wave' of delinquent acts, occurring in several cities, and including riotous behaviour, car chases and arson attacks. These events led to considerable public concern. Given their previous stance, the government then faced a major dilemma of how to respond. They needed new effective solutions which were not those they had previously condemned and were also, given the economic constraints, not too expensive.

The events of the summer of 1981 happened in urban areas where there were no facilities for young people. Remote central government in Paris did not seem to be the right agency to address and solve the problem. Instead, people from local communities of all ranks and roles were brought together to tackle the task.

THE MAYORS' COMMISSION

As a result, the Prime Minister Pierre Maurois set up a multi-party commission of mayors in 1982. They were charged with putting forward proposals to combat crime and the fear of crime. For the first time politicians from across the political spectrum were able to work together on this problem. The commission (known as the Bonnemaison Commission after its chairman) reported in late 1982. The main elements of this report are as follows:

1 The traditional approach of the police and the criminal justice system is inadequate to deal with crime.
2 The causes of crime are similar to those which cause suicides, drug and alcohol abuse, and mental illness. These causes include changes in family life, poor, segregated housing conditions, difficulties with social and work integration, breakdown in informal social controls and absence of leisure activities during the day. These causes are exacerbated by drugs, alcohol, increases in long-term unemployment and tempting goods.
3 To be effective, a policy to fight crime should be flexible, and adapted to local circumstances. It should link all the local partners: this should include several different parts of the administration such as the police, the judicial system, social service, public health, education, youth and sports, culture and housing; it also would include the elected officials such as the mayor and assistant mayor and representatives of the population such as the trade unions and the non-profit organisations (associations).

4 To be really effective in tackling crime, social prevention and law enforcement must be combined in a careful and controlled way. Its recommendations were guided by the need to establish local inter-agency co-operation and better use of current resources. As petty and common crime has not been stopped by the enforcement of laws and budgets could no longer be expanded, it was necessary to encourage the breakdown of bureaucratic barriers and encourage the reassessment of priorities to respond to crime problems more effectively at the local level. The commission's report puts forward solutions concerned with housing, training for employment and problems of young immigrants. However, it also stresses the need to have a crime policy that is both concerned with the enforcement of the law and with tackling the root causes of crime. The public should be involved, for instance, by working with young delinquents or with victims. This involvement will reduce public alienation from the system and combat the stereotypes generated by media sensationalism of events.

IMPLEMENTATION

A National Council on the Prevention of Crime (*Conseil National de Prévention de la Délinquance*) was created by a decree of 8 June 1983 under the chairmanship of the Prime Minister; on the departmental level, Departmental Councils for the Prevention of Crime were created for each Department, chaired by the Chief Administrator for the region (*Commissaire de la République*) and with the vice-chairman being the Chief Judicial Officer (*Procureur de la République*). Finally, the decree provided for a Communal Council for Prevention of Crime for any city that wanted to create one.

At each level, the councils have three bodies represented: the elected officials, representatives from the administration and representatives of citizen groups such as voluntary organisations and the unions. The mandate of the CNPD has developed over time. Initially it was expected to be aware of the trends in crime in France, to propose measures to the authorities that would prevent crime and reduce its effects, to examine the results from measures taken by ministers, and to promote a public better informed on these issues. When necessary, permanent working groups are created to deal with a special problem (drug addiction, community service orders, elderly people, young delinquents coming out of jail). For 1990 the budget of the CNPD was $14 million.

In 1983 there were Communal Councils in eighteen pilot cities drawn from those with different political parties in power. In 1984 there were forty-two pilot cities. There were 570 local crime prevention councils in France 1989. Of these approximately 180 have been set up for cities with populations of more than 30,000 (80 per cent of such cities). The decree establishing the CNPD makes the creation of the local city councils optional. There is thus an impressive level of involvement. Commentators suggest that roughly one-third of these councils exist little more than on paper, while one-third are working well and one-third are developing much better than the CNPD would have expected.

The local crime prevention council is chaired by the mayor with the local officials from the national ministries responsible for social affairs, schools, housing, sport, justice and police. It also includes other local councillors and municipal employees. Various local judges and non-profit organisations are involved in a consultative capacity and experts can be associated.

Most councils have a senior city official as the executive secretary, who plays an active part in preparing meetings and following through them to ensure that decisions are implemented. This official is undoubtedly essential to the success of the councils. In large cities a special council is often created in each district; this solution is generally considered as well-adapted for developing appropriate solutions to specific local problems.

Before the establishment of the councils, there had often been tensions between the police and the detached worker prevention programmes. The feeling had developed that the street programmes were not successful and tensions had arisen between the police and the social workers about specific offenders. The local crime prevention councils have become a focus for this work and a place where co-operation between police and social workers can develop.

The full councils meet once every couple of months. The tone of the meetings is collegial. Although administrators and politicians are official members, while private agencies are only consultative, everyone takes part in the discussions. They create a common ownership of crime.

The two objectives are intended, on the one hand, to provide more facilities and specialised services and, on the other, to offer suitable organised activities and a varied range of opportunities away from the home environment for young people living in deprived districts. Schemes must be aimed particularly at the social integration of those in greater difficulty and in greatest danger of becoming delinquent.

To take an example in the Department of 'Val-de-Marne' (south of Paris) during the summer of 1987, 76 programmes were organised for some 20,000 juveniles and young adults. Preference was given to programmes for people from 13 to 25 years old, especially those which aimed to develop social and cultural life in disadvantaged areas and were prepared by young inhabitants. Two of these programmes were reserved for prisoners in the local jail due for discharge.

Among these projects activities featured such as moto-cross, horse-riding, karting, aikido, ju-jitsu, making video films, exploring the home countries of migrant groups (Algeria, Portugal) evening activities (e.g. concerts, theatre), travel, and so on. During this period the numbers of young offenders coming to court were 40 per cent fewer than during the same period in 1981 when this type of programme did not exist.

INCREASING PUBLIC AWARENESS

Also associated with activity at the local level is the targeting of public opinion through information and awareness campaigns undertaken by the National Council; these include

1 Short programmes on television and at the cinema which spotlight the issues.
2 Videos on topics such as mediation in the community or young people's local councils.
3 A newsletter sent to all participants.
4 Local crime prevention weeks where officials and researchers can exchange views and publicise the programme.

WHAT ARE THE RESULTS?

It is too early to make a general assessment of the impact of the local city crime prevention councils. However, the national rate of crime per capita in France went down in 1985, 1986 and 1987, the drop of 8 per cent in 1986 being higher than any year since 1972. Further, comparisons between areas with a community crime prevention council and those without showed, for a range of common crimes, marginally larger reductions where the community crime prevention council existed, even though the latter tended to have higher rates of crime.

The 'summer programme' has also had an effect on crime during the summer months in central city areas by removing many of the young people most often involved in crime. While it may be only a short-term success, it is certainly a benefit. These projects do more than offer summer camps to those who would participate anyway, as they are specifically designed for those who would not normally join the equivalent of boys' clubs. Each summer an increasing number of regions and cities are covered by this programme. Moreover most of the activities developed for the summer are continued afterwards as local authorities and social workers are convinced of their value.

However, most of the projects are concerned with the medium-term prevention of crime. So helping North African children read better or developing better employment skills will increase self-esteem and reduce crime only over a number of years. So it is still too early to tell. Some of the French projects could appear to be part of general welfare provision rather than crime prevention. On closer inspection, the French projects tend to be close to 'secondary' crime prevention, that is focused on groups or situations that are pre-delinquent. Taking part in the councils also teaches the participants about the crime problem. In particular, the elected officials become more aware of the realities of crime and crime prevention than the 'sensational and exceptional myths' that sell media advertising. This new level of realism is also hard to measure.

The weak point is the failure to apply scientific knowledge in developing effective programmes. But local and governmental authorities have become more and more conscious of the necessity of improving the effectiveness of their approach by developing better and more relevant training for those working on the councils and by involving researchers and academics to assist the action.

This policy for prevention of crime was maintained by the right-wing government from 1986 to 1988. When the socialist government regained power some reorganisation was made at the national level. A large inter-ministerial delegation was created close to the Prime Minister to deal with all the problems related to cities: housing, urban design, social integration policies, inter-ethnic and inter-generation relationships and prevention of crime. This decision to regroup into the same national framework several policies for coping with urban development expresses the political will to work very deeply on the roots of crime, to prepare for the future conditions of life which no longer generate crime.

The 'French model' is apparently looked at with interest by a good number of foreign governments and policy-makers. In order to highlight, starting from this model, some suggestions for coping with the crime problem in a successful way, we could point out:

1. To be efficient, a policy against crime must be developed at the same time and in a coherent way at both national and local levels.
2. To reduce insecurity is not only to combat crime but also to prevent it.
3. Such a policy requires the involvement not only of police and the justice system but also above all of a wide range of social actors; an inter-agency approach is necessary.
4. Crime must be dealt with, at the local level, starting from its concrete reality and acting on its local roots. National policies must reserve space for local adaptations.
5. Politicians must cope with crime rather than exploit crime.
6. Such a crime prevention policy is necessarily a medium- and long-term policy.

Representatives of several important European cities decided, with the approbation of the Council of Europe to create in November 1987 a 'European Forum of Cities for Urban Security' organising co-operation and exchange on the difficult problem of fighting and preventing crime. In October 1989 an international conference was held in Montreal co-organised by the US Conference of Mayors, the Canadian Federation of Municipalities and the European Forum. About 1,000 representatives of regions of the world were present and adopted by consensus a programme modelled on the French policies.

© 1991 Marie-Pierre de Liège

Chapter ten

A touch of discipline

Accountability and discipline in prison systems in western Europe[1]

Jon Vagg

Prisons have rules, and when prisoners break them they get punished. It is not of course as simple as that. Prison officers have to realise that some rule has been, or is being, broken. They must make a report to senior staff and/or the governor. In some countries they might make a report not because a prisoner has done something specific but because he or she is generally unco-operative. The governor is expected to follow laid-down procedures. The outcome may be, as it is phrased in England and Wales, an 'award'. Other consequences, such as transfer to another institution, might also follow; the disciplinary record might be taken into account at future stages in the inmate's 'prison career', for example in decisions about parole. Finally, and most crucially from the point of view of accountability, the inmate may have the opportunity to challenge the governor's decision, which might then be reduced or set aside, and perhaps even some form of compensation given – the specific arrangements, of course, varying across the four countries with which I shall be concerned: England and Wales, France, the Federal Republic of Germany (FRG) and the Netherlands.

In England and Wales, questions have been raised about the ways in which prison discipline operates. The reasons for raising them are somewhat Anglo-centric, and explained in the body of this chapter (see also Morgan *et al.* 1985; Zellick 1981, 1982). But in essence, they are first, how far are prison governors accountable to others for the disciplinary procedures and the punishments they impose on inmates? Second, and more specifically, what is the relationship between disciplinary proceedings, other administrative actions which might be construed, whatever their objectives, as 'punishments in effect', and the possibilities for prisoners to seek remedies against such proceedings and action?

I have been studying prison accountability in four countries which present a range of practices.[2] The intention was not to make direct comparisons between countries, nor to discover good things abroad that could be imported to England and Wales. In Britain, and probably elsewhere too, penologists study a prison system shaped by parochial values, assumptions and experiences. Comments on the system tend to draw on those same factors that have shaped it. Looking at a range of systems gives, even at its most limited, a broader understanding of how important or unimportant those factors are. Beyond that, even the most cursory examination of systems other than our own is able to illuminate parochial debates by giving us a sense of how usual, or how unique, are our own problems and our assumptions about their nature.

The next section of this chapter reviews the disciplinary processes and the use of sanctions in the four countries. The two following sections each address one of the questions posed above, and the fourth tries to draw together the strands of data and description into some conclusions.

FORMAL DISCIPLINARY SANCTIONS

In England and Wales, the Prison Rules group together in Rule 47 all those things for which disciplinary hearings and punishments are possible. In the other three countries the responsibilities and obligations of inmates are scattered through a range of clauses in their penal codes and prison rules. However, the rules in all countries cover the same general ground, with broad requirements to obey officers and to obey specific rules for the particular establishment, and prohibitions of disorderly conduct and noisy behaviour.[3] Convicted prisoners are required to work satisfactorily. There are differences in the kinds of goods and services prisoners are entitled to have and receive, and consequently in those which are unauthorised and could form the basis of a disciplinary offence. All sets of rules contain one or more 'etcetera clauses', rules which may be applied where none of the more specific prohibitions covers the situation.

The 'hearing of first instance' in all four countries is before the prison governor or deputy. It is usually brief, and takes place the day after the alleged offence. There is a broad similarity between England and Wales, France and the Federal Republic of Germany in at least some aspects of natural justice; prisoners should be given a written statement of the charge prior to the hearing and have the opportunity to present their side of the affair. In England and Wales, the hearing is formally divided into two sections, the first concerned with guilt or innocence and the second with mitigation and punishment. There is sometimes, though not always, a short written statement from staff who know the prisoner which is presented as mitigation. In the FRG the hearing may, and in France must, involve senior staff and sometimes also social work personnel (and in the FRG the prison doctor) who advise the governor, although in neither case is it necessary for the officer who reported the infraction to be present, as in England and Wales.

In England and Wales and in France, the formality of the proceedings is reinforced by the use of a special adjudication room for the hearing. In the Netherlands, the fact that the governor or an assistant governor conducts the disciplinary procedure at the prisoner's cell door gives greater scope for informality. The statement of the punishment is, however, more precise. Governors are expected to include on the form authorising the punishment not only the date but also the time at which the punishment takes effect, for example 'confined to cell 10am 2.4.86 to 10am 9.4.86'; and the form has, printed on it, a note that the complaints committee of the prison will hear any appeal against the hearing.

Three points emerge from a study of the formal sanctions available in the countries (see Table 10.1). First, there is a difference of approach between England and Wales and the other countries. France, the FRG and the Netherlands allow governors to use only confinement to cell or to a punishment cell as a punishment. In England and Wales this power is very restricted at governor level and the major power to punish resides in the removal of remission of sentence. In England and Wales remission is calculated on reception into prison and an 'earliest date of release' set. Governors can then withdraw remission which is in effect already granted. In France remission is a judicial responsibility and in the FRG it does not exist. Only the Netherlands has a roughly comparable system, in as much as what was until 1986 a parole system then became in effect a system of remission, with inmates released automatically unless the governor recommended that the Ministry of Justice review the case. Second, while all four countries have two levels of response – the governor and the

Table 10.1 Disciplinary punishments available in England and Wales, the Netherlands, France and the Federal Republic of Germany

England and Wales

1 caution
2 forfeiture/postponement of privileges (e.g. purchase of items in prison) maximum [governor 28 days, Board of Visitors (BoV) any period]
3 exclusion from associated work, maximum [governor 14 days, BoV 56 days]
4 stoppage of earnings, maximum [governor 28 days BoV 56 days]
5 cellular confinement, maximum [governor 28 days, BoV 56 days]
6 forfeiture of remission, maximum [governor 28 days, BoV 180 days except no limit for charges of gross personal violence, mutiny]
7 forfeiture for any period of the right to have articles (e.g. books, newspapers, writing materials, etc.)[a]
8 forfeiture for any period of the right to wear own clothing if guilty of escape/attempt escape[a]

The Netherlands

1 confinement to isolation cell, maximum 2 weeks
2 confinement to own or other cell, maximum 2 weeks (may be a confinement only for certain hours of the day)
3 reprimand

France[b]

1 warning
2 declassification at work (if offence committed there)
3 removal of privilege to buy beer, cider, toiletries, etc., to receive items from outside prison, or other privileges, no limit of time
4 removal of privilege of use of individual radio
5 removal of privilege of open visits (if offence committed there)
6 punishment cell, maximum 45 days.

Federal Republic of Germany

1 warning
2 limitation/deprivation of prison moneys and purchases, maximum 3 months
3 limitation/deprivation of reading matter maximum 2 weeks; of radio/TV maximum 3 months; of both together maximum 2 weeks
4 limitation/deprivation of free time activity/group events, maximum 3 months
5 separate accommodation during free time, maximum 4 weeks
6 deprivation of daily leave (if applicable), maximum 1 week
7 deprivation of work/activity, maximum 4 weeks
8 limitation of communication (except urgent matters), maximum 3 months
9 punishment cell, maximum 4 weeks

Notes: [a]Unconvicted prisoners only
[b]Payment for damage to materials may also be demanded but is not a sanction

Sources: England and Wales: Prison Rules 50, 51, 52
Netherlands: Ministerie van Justitie (no date)
France: Code de Procedure Penale, Art D250
FRG: St VollzG s103(1)

courts, with the latter in practice rarely used – the English prison system has available to it an intermediate step, the Boards of Visitors.[4] The boards constitute a means of discipline readily available to the governor within the institution and operating under the Prison Rules. If one phrases it in this way, the third point is that English prisoners are far and away the most vulnerable to very severe internal sanctions indeed. If one stresses the Boards' independence, the point is simply that recourse to an independent disciplinary process with powers to use severe sanctions is far more common in England and Wales than elsewhere.

Maximum penalties are one thing; usual practice is another. It is difficult to piece together a comprehensive picture, largely due to differences in the information collected internally in the prison systems and in that which is published. For the most formal system, the English, quite a lot of data are published. For the least formal system, the Dutch, the department itself does not collect comprehensive data. However, it seems (see Table 10.2) that England and Wales and the Netherlands both use punishments extensively, with the Dutch using confinement to cell more often since fewer types of sanctions are available. In England and Wales it is common for two types of punishments to be imposed simultaneously, while cellular confinement is often served in a punishment cell. In the Netherlands prisoners are usually confined in their own cells, and retain personal possessions and televisions rented from the prison authorities. On these grounds one can say that the punishments in the Netherlands are much less stringent. In France and the FRG the overall level of punishment is much less, though in France the punishment cell is used in over half of all cases and usually for eight to fifteen days rather than the two or three often found in England (Ministère de la Justice 1987). Unfortunately no comparable data on the length of cellular confinement are available from the FRG. Finally, the punishment 'norms' seem to vary more between institutions within countries more than they do between the countries. This seems likely to reflect – and officials, staff and inmates interviewed all agree on this – a differential 'opportunity structure' of offending within different establishments and also a difference in staff expectations, with some prisons being more controlled by formal disciplinary means than others.

Table 10.2 Extent of use of disciplinary punishments in England and Wales, the Netherlands, France and the Federal Republic of Germany

England and Wales: offences punished per 100 population (to nearest 10)

1985 = 170 1986 = 170

Variation in rate per 100 prisoners, by type of prison (selected) 1986

	Male	*Female*
remand centres	280	300
local prisons	110	330
closed training	130	390
closed youth custody	320	910

The Netherlands: data available for selected establishments and sample periods only

Type of prison	*Sample period*	*Rate per 100 prisoners p/a*
open, for 14dy–6m sentences	209 days, 1987	179
closed, long term	– all 1986	90
	– 181 days, 1987	37
closed, remand house	all 1986	286
closed, female	181 days, 1987	155

France: sanctions per 100 prisoners 1985–6

1985 = 100 (indexed against 1.1.85 population)
101 (indexed against 1.1.86 population)
1986 = 100 (indexed against 1.1.86 population)
89 (indexed against 1.1.87 population)

Sanctions by type of prison	>	Maisons d' ârret =101
1985 per 100 prisoners	>	Maisons centrales = 73
(against 1.1.86 population)	>	Centres de detention 84

Federal Republic of Germany: sanctions per 100 prisoners, by Land (selected) 1986

State	*Sanctions per 100 prisoners*	*Remarks*
Bremen	26.5	smallest system, lowest sanction rate
Nordrhein-Westfalia	72.0	largest system, av. sanction rate
Saarland	90.0	2nd smallest system, highest sanction rate
Federal	64.8	

Sources: England and Wales: Prison Statistics 1986
Netherlands: JV
France: Ministère de la Justice 1987
FRG: Länder returns to Federal Ministry 1986

FORMAL DISCIPLINE AND ACCOUNTABILITY

How far are prison governors accountable for the disciplinary procedures and the punishments they impose on inmates? My data cover four aspects of this question: the routine monitoring of governors' decisions, procedures in the case of serious incidents, the prosecution of inmates in the courts, and inmate-initiated complaints and reviews of disciplinary decisions.

What kinds of controls and constraints are imposed on governors by departmental monitoring mechanisms? In England and Wales all records of disciplinary hearings are forwarded to regional offices and an assistant regional director scrutinises them to ensure that no unsafe decisions have been taken. Nationally there are in the region of 72,000 forms submitted each year, with four assistant regional directors, who also have other tasks, to scrutinise them. In France, the regional director's office receives notification of all disciplinary punishments for the region, and the *juge de l'application des peines* (or 'JAP')[5] for the prison receives notification of all the cases in his or her prison. With this two-tier system, nine regional directorates and around 42,000 to 43,000 cases each year, there is a greater possibility for internal monitoring, though I have no figures for the number of punishments altered or withdrawn as a result. The JAPs have no power to alter punishments but are entitled to raise cases they think are problematic with the governor and/or the regional director. My interviews with governors suggest that this action is very rarely taken. In neither the FRG nor the Netherlands does there seem to be any routine monitoring of disciplinary decisions. Accountability from this source is, therefore, very weak in all four countries.

All prison systems provide special instructions to governors concerning serious incidents. In essence, they are reported to the regional or central administration which then determines how the matter will be dealt with. To this extent, accountability is less of an issue than control. However, in practice, one can find in all countries differences between governors as to the interpretation of 'serious'. And, as governors and ministerial officials in both the FRG and the Netherlands noted, there are differences between prisons in what one governor called 'the grasp of the administration' – that is in just how interested the adminstration is in what happens in a particular prison. Where 'the grasp' is tight, governors may feel less able to avoid reporting matters. But the grasp tends to be tighter in higher-security prisons, and during periods of widespread inmate unrest. This aspect of accountability is, from the point of view of discipline, not unlike a colander.

One further aspect of centralised control has to do with the possibility of prosecuting the inmate in court rather than (or as well as) giving an internal sanction. Three quick comments are pertinent. First, in England and Wales the existence of the Boards of Visitors offers a 'middle way'. Prison Rules 51 and 52 provide for certain kinds of charges to be heard only by Boards of Visitors, and for the size of adjudicating panels and the number of magistrates sitting on them to be increased when dealing with very serious charges. Second, the prison authorities refer cases to the police and/or prosecuting bodies; they do not undertake prosecutions themselves. And between the prisons, headquarters staff and prosecution authorities, confusion is possible. France provides the clearest example. Menard and Meurs (1984) note that any serious incident affecting discipline or security should be reported to the *Préfet* and the *Procureur* as well as the Regional Director and the central administration, while in the case of assaults on staff, different offices within the administration appear to use different criteria in assessing the seriousness of the 'incident' and confusion could arise over the desirability of pressing for a court prosecution. Third, differences exist in the extent to which inmates are prosecuted, and not in the direction one might suppose. In England and Wales, even though most serious cases are heard by Boards of Visitors, statistics for Prison Department South West Region indicate twenty-two such prosecutions in 1985 and twenty-seven in 1986 (the regional average daily population was about 7,500). Complete data for France are not available. But Menard and Meurs (1984) noted a national total of forty-nine aggressions prosecuted in 1982 of which, after allowing for those cases not proceeded with, twenty-seven resulted in further sentences. The year-end penal population in that year was about 34,500. And, according to prison governors and ministry staff whom I interviewed, prosecution for other matters seems rare although no figures are available. In the Netherlands, interestingly because the level of punishment available internally is so low, none of the ministry staff I spoke to (including those in the legal section) and none of the governors could recall a case ever having been prosecuted in the courts. The FRG data are, unfortunately, entirely lacking. The files do not appear to be collated into a statistical form.

Turning to the complaints systems, the single most important point is that complaints are dealt with only after the measure complained of has already taken effect, and that remedies are similarly *post hoc.* None the less, the four systems show great differences in the extent to which disciplinary matters are partitioned off as matters of special significance. Prisoners in France may complain about disciplinary decisions, directly or via their lawyer, to the administration. They may also write, or ask their lawyer to write, to the JAP, though this is less an avenue of complaint than an opportunity to explain their case in the hope that the JAP will disregard the infraction when considering home leave, remission and so forth. There is currently no means of court review of an internal disciplinary punishment; the civil courts are constitutionally precluded from hearing such cases, and the administrative courts have not accepted any jurisdiction in this area. One case is, as I write, under way which challenges this position and may yet open up the possibility of legal review. Inmates in England and Wales have the possibility of writing a petition to the administration complaining about the decision (guilt or level of punishment). No precise figures are available, but the Prison Department estimates that around 5 per cent of petitions concerning discipline result in a remission or mitigation of punishment although for 1988 the figure 'blipped' nearer to 10 per cent (source: Prison Department). In contrast to France, however, inmates do have a judicial means of redress, *so far as the correctness of procedure* is concerned. A large body of case law now covers areas such as the evidence necessary to secure a finding of guilt, and the circumstances under which prisoners should have the possibility of legal representation at the hearings (though requests for it are still rare; in 1986, of 3,765 Boards of Visitors adjudications, legal representation was requested in only 183 cases and granted in only 59). Most of the cases concern Boards of Visitors adjudications; and though the recent cases of *Leech* and *Prevot* have opened governors' hearings to judicial review, we have yet to see the effects of this. The courts have not – yet – seen fit to review the justness of the level of punishment and this can be pursued only through internal petitions.

In both the FRG and the Netherlands, complaints about disciplinary decisions are treated in the same way as complaints about any other area of prison life. In the FRG complaints may be made to a branch of the criminal courts, the *Strafvollstreckungskammer* (in some Länder this may be done directly, in others the complaint must be aired with the ministry first). If satisfaction is not received there, the matter may be taken to the next higher court, the *Oberlandesgericht* (OLG). The procedure at both levels is almost entirely written, and complaints are accepted only where it is alleged that the law (usually the *Strafvollzugsgesetz* or *StVollzG*) rather than administrative rules have been breached.[6] There are no separate figures for complaints concerning disciplinary offences, but overall success rates for complaints are low; around 2–3 per cent in the lower courts (Kaiser *et al.* 1983) and around 5 per cent at the lower and higher levels combined (Feest 1988). In the Netherlands a new complaints system came into operation in 1977, revolving around independent boards with memberships including, for example, housewives, businessmen, lawyers and academics. Complaints go first to the institutional-level *Commissie van Toezicht* (CvT), from where they can be appealed by either inmate or governor to the national *Centrale Raad van Advies* (CRvA). In 1986 just over 16 per cent of all complaints to the CvTs were found grounded, and of the one quarter or so finding their way to the higher-level CRvA, about 27 per cent of inmate appeals were upheld (though governors had a higher success rate, with 65 per cent of their appeals being upheld). Of the four countries, then, prisoners in the Dutch system have the best chance of a successful challenge to a disciplinary measure although by the time of the decision the punishment will already have been served. To deal with this, the CvTs and the CRvA are empowered to grant compensation, usually in the form of extra exercise, extra visits, or in some cases a small amount of money.

It is worth pausing, before moving on to a discussion of 'informal' sanctions, to take stock of the situation with regard to formal disciplinary measures. Five main points have emerged so far. First, in principle governors have less discretion where offences are more serious, at least so far as the handling of the cases is concerned. But the extent to which practice corresponds to theory varies with the predilections of the governor and the preoccupations of the regional and central administration. Second, the types of punishments vary between England and Wales and the other countries, with England and Wales devolving substantial powers of loss of remission to governors and other countries relying on the use of confinement to cell and the punishment cells. Third, the English three-tier system ought to mean that fewer cases are sent to the courts than in the other countries, but the indications available suggest that this is probably not so. Fourth, internal controls on disciplinary decisions are in most 'normal' cases, weak or non-existent, and perforce the major avenue of accountability lies to the courts and the complaints systems. And fifth, there is, if anything, a correlation between the severity of punishment that can be given and a lack of means of redress. The Netherlands appears to have the most informal approach, the least severe sanctions and the complaints system offering the best chance of overturning disciplinary decisions. France gives its governors extensive powers and provides no opportunity of redress outside the organisational hierarchy. England is the odd one out; accountability for disciplinary matters has become increasingly judicialised though only in relation to procedure.

PUNISHMENT IN EFFECT?

The extent of the 'alternative disciplinary system' became an issue in England and Wales when the Tarrant court decision allowed inmates access to legal representation in Board of Visitors disciplinary hearings (the precise nature of the right is still controversial; see Fitzgerald 1985; Morgan and Macfarlane 1985; Quinn 1985). It was suggested to the subsequent Departmental Committee (Home Office 1985b) that any increase in the formality of the 'official' system, lengthy delays prior to hearings, or large proportions of technical acquittals would shift the nature of control towards an 'alternative disciplinary system' comprising administrative segregation, transfers, security re-categorisation, removal of privileges and so forth (Morgan *et al.* 1985; POA 1984). Some parts of this system require action by the prison governor; others can be deployed by staff on the landings; and the system quite clearly operates alongside, as well as independently of, formal disciplinary procedures – as when an inmate is not only given a formal punishment but also transferred, perhaps repeatedly – a process known in England as 'ghosting', in the Netherlands as 'going on the carousel'. What factors are likely to determine the extent to which administrative actions rather than (or as well as) formal disciplinary measures are likely to be used?

First, the idea that formal discipline is a special area that should be cordoned off from other administrative actions is virtually non-existent outside England and Wales, and it seems to exist there largely because of the success with which inmates have challenged Board of Visitors disciplinary hearings in the courts, thereby suggesting that formally determined punishments for serious offences are especially vulnerable to judicial review (Richardson 1985). In the other countries, formal disciplinary matters are as vulnerable (or as little vulnerable) to inmate actions as are any other areas about which inmates may complain or litigate. And so there may be little motive for governors to try to circumvent the formal procedures. This does not mean, of course, that they will not use segregation or set in motion transfers as an adjunct to a formal punishment; simply that, save in the English case, decisions about punishment, segregation and transfer are all subject to a more or less similar degree of accountability, whatever degree that might be in the individual country.

In practice, it seems likely that high or low rates for formal punishment and high or low rates for other measures are heavily influenced by the 'prison management culture' of a prison system or the institutional culture of a prison. Data from the eleven prison systems of the FRG illustrate this. These data, comprising returns to the Federal Justice Ministry from the individual Länder and relating to 1986, are not detailed enough to show variations between individual establishments; nor are they broken down by categories of prisoner. And they must be interpreted with care since some Länder have only one or two prisons while others have thirty or forty, so that the basis from which the overall rate is derived varies substantially by Land. However, a comparison of the use of 'special measures' – mainly isolation – and disciplinary rates indicates that all four possibilities given by low or high rates of discipline and of special measures exist in practice. Hamburg and Bayern both use disciplinary measures extensively (82.6 and 80 punishments per 100 inmates respectively in 1986). Hamburg used 'special measures' almost as frequently (84.1 per 100 inmates for the year) while Bayern used almost none (3.4 per 100 inmates). Berlin and Hessen both used disciplinary measures quite rarely (31.4 and 30.5 per 100 inmates) but in 1986 the former used 'special measures' almost two and a half times more frequently (44.7 per 100 inmates as opposed to 18.4). Admittedly Hamburg and Berlin are smallish systems, perhaps with less stable year-on-year rates. Yet these figures suggest that there is no general 'trade-off' between the two areas of discipline and segregation or other special measures.

A second factor influencing the balance between disciplinary and other administrative procedures may be the physical arrangements in the prisons and, where they exist, capacity problems. In the Dutch open prison I visited, the majority of drugs infractions had until recently simply resulted in segregation pending transfer to a closed prison; that is, in effect, an administrative rather than formal disciplinary measure. Governor grades frankly stated that they did not have the facilities to impose lengthy periods in the punishment cells (of which they had three). Thus as one governor said:

> If it's a serious threat to personnel they go for two weeks to Maastricht or Veenhuizen [prisons with special isolation units]. If I want to punish for 14 days I will send inmates there because I can't afford the space in my own establishment. We don't give suspended disciplinary punishments as such. It depends on the use of *Strafzelle.* If we need it and it is occupied we will conditionally release those in it. But this is not often used.

However, capacity problems in the closed prisons had begun to mean that inmates would wait for long periods in segregation before transfer was possible. In consequence, the governor had begun to use punishments of one or two days in the punishment cell as an alternative to transfer. Disciplinary measures had thus come to be applied instead of administrative measures because the latter had become impracticable.

Third, some governors would claim that using administrative rather than disciplinary measures is not always to the inmates' disadvantage. In one establishment in the FRG, the governor appointed in 1978–9 differed in his approach from his predecessor. He decided that refusals of inmates to work would no longer be treated as disciplinary matters but that the inmate would, instead, simply be locked in his cell. He relied on boredom and the loss of earnings for the day as *de facto* sanctions. The rate of disciplinary hearings per 100 prisoners per year fell drastically: from 157 prior to his arrival to 55 in 1979, and for all subsequent years fluctuating between about 42 and 18. Equally, Dutch prison governors defended the transfer of inmates to another wing of the prison or to another prison if, for example, they had assaulted staff, on the grounds that this prevented the use of more severe informal sanctions by staff.

But fourth, administrative changes in particular relating to security may be felt by inmates as, in effect, group punishments for actions carried out by small numbers of inmates. One inmate in a Dutch maximum-security prison had this to say about changes in the prison regime following an escape:

> They say that you don't get a punishment for escaping . . . but in October '86 [after an inmate escaped] the regime gets tougher. There is a strict group-separation of side [i.e. wing] A and B. No walking around anymore. In the evening-hours no sports. The groups have to use the telephone separately. One group in the cells, the others telephoning, washing, taking a shower. One group evening recreation the others not, so recreation is halved. These changes are probably due to the fact that the staff couldn't control it anymore. The prisoners had too much influence.

The discussion so far has largely set aside the issue of informal sanctions applied at the level of the officers, though this is clearly a matter of some importance.

In England and Wales and the Netherlands, staff had wide discretion over many of the more trivial day-to-day aspects of prisoners' lives – and in the Netherlands, where inmates have a wider range of privileges, staff had a proportionately wider sphere of discretion. This could be exercised in a wide variety of ways, from delays in opening cell doors to telling prisoners to 'fuck off' when they request something (this last is also reported in Maguire and Vagg 1984) or (in some Dutch prisons) being uncooperative about arrangements for inmate phone calls. The wider range of privileges also, incidentally, gives Dutch staff a wider range of positive measures: where else would one see a prison officer helping an inmate to repair his Walkman? However, informal sanctions were not necessarily easy or straightforward to apply. Staff in both countries pointed out that the kinds of inmates who might be considered targets for such actions were, anyway, the uncooperative prisoners who were likely to make complaints about such things and who (in England and Wales) typically regarded the internal complaints procedures as valueless and who would thus go to their lawyers for remedy. To apply informal sanctions to such inmates, staff said, would be invite further and perhaps legal trouble. This does not mean that such things did not happen; but in interviews, and despite prodding, inmates said it did not happen much and that they were surprised at how little evidence there was of such treatment given the obvious potential for it. McDermott and King (1988), in a study of some English prisons, use a 'game' metaphor to suggest that informal sanctions and inmate strategies and responses do not exist in isolation, but are part of a longer-running struggle for self-identity and control in an environment where inmates are virtually powerless. It seems likely that such games are played in general at a fairly low intensity, but at some places and times, or with some inmates, at a much higher level and maybe for higher stakes.

Dutch and English inmates in my own study were less concerned about deliberately applied informal sanctions than they were about inconsistency among staff in applying formal ones. In one prison, inmates said that some staff would facilitate swapping cassette tapes by taking them to and from other inmates (in principle prohibited by Prison Rules and Standing Orders), while others would 'go by the book' and make out disciplinary reports where inmates were found in possession of each others' tapes or trying to swap them. And some staff were said to allow or report such things depending on their mood.

In the FRG and France both staff and inmates said that the staff were controlled to a very high degree by senior staff to whom almost any decision of consequence to inmates needed to be referred. Inmates did complain about, for example, the range of goods in the prison canteen and about decisions of the governor; but they were agreed that any informal sanctions by basic-grade staff were most unlikely. In France, inmates said that staff were even afraid to open cell doors for inmates to collect items at times when the inmates were supposed to be out of their cells. However, if informal sanctions were rare, manipulation of the formal disciplinary system could and did occur: 'After the first or second time, punishment is more frequent, they search you out, provoke you; not systematically, but for several inmates it has happened' (inmate, French *maison centrale*).

FINDING A CONTEXT

I started this chapter with two questions: how far are prison governors accountable to others for the disciplinary procedures and the punishments they impose on inmates? What is the relationship between disciplinary proceedings, administrative 'punishments in effect', and grievance procedures? The answers are: they are as much, or more usually as little, accountable for discipline as they are for any of the alternatives they might use, except in England where inmate rights have grown lopsidedly; and while 'alternative' disciplinary measures are possible, they do not really constitute a system so much as an adjunct to the formal processes. What is more important is the extent to which changes in regimes feel like collective punishments, and the extent to which staff are inconsistent in making reports which result in formal sanctions.

But like most answers, these raise further questions about the context in which prison discipline is applied and in which it will develop. Let me, by way of a conclusion, quickly point out two areas which impinge on prison discipline and which may affect its future development in the four countries.

The first, *prison conditions*, is related to inmate perceptions of what might constitute a 'punishment in effect'. In England and Wales and France, prison populations have been increasing rapidly; in the Netherlands there has been pressure to review the policy of only one inmate per cell. Dutch regimes were, in 1986–7, coming under budgetary pressure and the amount of time spent in workshops had been cut shortly before. In England and Wales perhaps the most pithy comment is that made by King and McDermott (1989), that regimes in high-security, long-term prisons today have deteriorated in many respects to resemble those of local, short-term and remand prisons fifteen or twenty years ago. Today's inmates were probably not, on the whole, in prison twenty years ago. But they have another way of assessing regimes; the comparisons between the privileges and facilities open to them and those open to others – for example, long-term as opposed to short-term prisoners, convicted as against remand, ordinary inmates as against those they know the staff consider troublesome and so on. If – or more likely as – regimes deteriorate, inmates may increasingly see themselves in the kind of regime that formerly applied only to the least-privileged inmates. If, or more likely when, they define their situation as one of being 'punished for nothing', inmate unrest will emerge increasingly strongly.

Second is the issue of *inmate rights*. A quick survey of inmate rights suggests that across all four countries, most are more accurately described as privileges or else are so heavily qualified as to give very little to the inmate (Vagg and Vossen 1988). And most are rights in relation to procedures rather than substantive matters such as prison conditions. None the less their scope and permissiveness has gradually increased in the last fifteen or so years. They will probably, if gradually, continue to increase. The problem in England and Wales has been that rights have developed faster in relation to discipline than in any other area. In the FRG and the Netherlands, rights have developed in relation to complaints and are more or less equally applicable to any of the things governors might wish to do to or with inmates. The development of rights as it has occurred in England and Wales has imposed a strain on the prison system, in that governors have been exposed to very dissimilar measures of accountability for discipline as against other, 'administrative', decisions: hence the concerns that prompted this chapter. England and Wales need, quite badly, either a revision of the law concerning prisons and in particular inmate complaints, or an increasing willingness of the courts to accept that they should review decisions other than disciplinary ones. It would be foolish to deny the 'blind spots' in the other administrations, or to deny that increasing rights will cause strains in their prisons. But their attention to complaints procedures in the past, and their refusal to mark out prison discipline as somehow an area apart from others, should ease their growing pains in the future.

POSTSCRIPT

Since this chapter was written, the Prison Rules (England and Wales) have been revised. The amendments, which came into force on 1 April 1989, made a number of important changes to the disciplinary processes. First, the euphemism 'award' has been abandoned in favour of the straightforward term 'punishment'. Second, the categorisation of some offences as 'especially grave' has been done away with and the subsections of Rule 47, defining the various offences, have been renumbered. Offences of 'mutiny' and 'gross personal violence' have also been 'taken off the books'. The requirements for Boards of Visitors to include larger numbers of magistrates when hearing certain cases has therefore also been superseded. Third, the maximum penalty available to Boards of Visitors has been reduced to 120 days' loss of remission. Some new administrative practices have also been implemented, of which the most important are that 'governors' adjudications' may now be delegated below the level of deputy governor (who is now designated 'Head of Custody'), and that records of disciplinary hearings are no longer sent for scrutiny to Regional offices, but are overseen as part of another internal inspection process. I am grateful to the Prison Department for keeping me informed of these developments.

© 1991 Jon Vagg

Chapter eleven

Conflict resolution between victims and offenders in Austria and in the Federal Republic of Germany

Christa Pelikan

The conflict resolution schemes I am going to present are all located within the juvenile justice system. It is significant and important to keep in mind that juvenile justice and the juvenile court traditionally serve as a field of experimentation for the criminal justice system in general. Reforms and new ideas grow and flourish easily there as they do not seem to pose the same kind of threat for the established system as elsewhere, youth itself being associated with change and with hope for the future. Indeed, new ideas do sometimes make progress even in the grim and hardened field of criminal justice. This has been the case with conflict resolution, the initiative taken with juveniles, which I shall describe in this chapter, having stimulated discussion about starting a project with adult offenders. This could be referred to as the avantgarde or *Vorreiterstellung* of juvenile justice.

First, I shall provide some background information about the way the Austrian juvenile justice system works and about the profile of juvenile delinquency in Austria. Later in the chapter, I shall give a rough outline of the corresponding features of juvenile justice in the Federal Republic of Germany (FRG).

As elsewhere juvenile offenders come under a special law which in Austria is the *Jugendgerichtsgesetz* (Juvenile Justice Law) which was first introduced in 1928. 'Juveniles' according to this law are persons between 14 and 19 years of age, 19-year-olds having been included in this category only since the new Juvenile Justice Law of 1988. Criminal procedure in juvenile justice matters, however, is the same as that for adults. This means juveniles are subject to one of the central guiding principles of the Austrian Code of Criminal Procedure, namely the *Legalitätsprinzip* (the 'principle of legality'), as opposed to the *Opportunitätsprinzip* (the 'principle of discretion'). According to the principle of legality the public prosecutor's office is theoretically granted no discretion to decide whether or not the public interest would be served by instituting prosecution proceedings in a specific case, but rather is obliged to bring to trial every offence which comes to its attention. According to the principle of discretion, however, the public prosecutor's office would be authorised, within the framework of applicable law, to exercise discretion in deciding whether or not the interest of criminal justice would be served by pursuing a specific offence through the courts.

Additionally it is a peculiarity of criminal law in Austria that there exists almost no prosecution by private petition of the injured party. The prosecutor's office thus has a kind of monopoly and at the same time a strictly defined duty to prosecute the criminal acts that come to its attention.

As a consequence, there is a wide range of petty offences reported to the police and brought to the notice of the prosecutor which subsequently lead to indictment and to criminal trial, irrespective of the injured party's interest or wishes concerning such a procedure. This is particularly the case for the vast number of offences that stem from the ownership and use of motor vehicles for acts of vandalism and disturbing the peace and for brawls and assaults by youths and groups of youths. Once the machine of the judiciary is set into motion, the role of the victim is reduced to that of an uninvolved bystander or of a witness who has to contribute to the task of finding the truth and assessing the guilt of the offender.

Although state prosecutors still subscribe to the kind of reasoning underlying the principle of legality, namely that the crime represents an injury not only to the individual but also to the collective, they are also aware of the fact that the cost of mobilising the complicated apparatus of the court and of the jury is unreasonably high.

One has to add that the profile of juvenile delinquency in Austria is characterised by the kind of minor offences mentioned above and also that the rate of offences reported to the police per 100,000 persons in the 14 to 18 age group has been decreasing. In this group 3,235 offences per 100,000 population were reported for offences in 1985, 3,291 in 1986 and 3,010 in 1987. In the FRG we find a rate of 3,963 in 1985, of 3,941 in 1986 and of 3,990 in 1987. (Up to 1975 the term 'youth' applied to 14–18-year-old 'juveniles' and to 18–21-year-old 'young adults'.) The same tendency holds true for sentencing practice, especially prison sentences. In 1985 there was a daily average prison population of 125 young people between 14 and 18 years of age in all of Austria's prisons, this representing a rate of 23 per 100,000 juveniles. (In the FRG in 1984 this rate was 18.5 per 100,000 for the same age group.)

These figures indicate a widespread distrust of incarceration as a means of dealing with events defined as 'criminal'. Almost unanimously judges and prosecutors have for some time come to agree that prison confinement for juveniles has achieved nothing in the way of resocialisation and indeed that it is in many ways counterproductive. This change of attitude started somewhat earlier in the FRG than in Austria and has resulted in a considerable drop in rates of imprisonment for juveniles (Cremer-Schäfer 1988; 78–84). In Austria, juvenile offenders benefited from the reform of the Penal Law Code in 1975, the number of sentences and the numbers sent to custody having decreased since then. In the early 1970s the sentencing rate had been about 2,000 per 100,000 juveniles and the rate of 14–18-year-olds imprisoned had been slightly over 100 per 100,000 per year.

Whenever a judge is of the opinion that care and rehabilitation is required, he or she may make use of the probation service which was established in 1964, the Probation Service law having been enacted in 1969. The probation service is another of the peculiarities of the Austrian system and is a progressive element within the criminal justice system of the country. It is not a state agency in the strict sense. This is particularly remarkable in view of the strong tradition of centralised provision of welfare services by the state; indeed state institutions hold a virtual monopoly. The *Verein für Bewährungshilfe und Soziale Arbeit* (Probation Service and Social Work Association) is not a branch of the court but is organised as a private association subsidised by the Ministry of Justice. Because of its independence, the service exercises considerable discretion in deciding about organisational matters and the methods of working with its clients.

Returning to the instruments of criminal law, there remain a vast number of petty offences to be dealt with. Until recently, the instruments provided by the Austrian Juvenile Justice Law consisted of the suspended sentence, the fine (conditional or unconditional), admonition by the judge or the conditional custodial sentence resulting from fully fledged jury proceedings. These measures were felt to be inappropriate – something like the proverbial shooting of sparrows with cannonballs. That is where innovative thinking about a new Juvenile Criminal Law started from.

New instruments have been created. A provision exists to drop an indictment after conflict resolution has succeeded or at least an effort made by the youth has been recorded by the court (paragraph 7 of the *Jugendgerichtsgesetz* [JGG] 1988). Conflict resolution can also be initiated by the judge (if the state prosecutor has decided to prosecute) who has the power to suspend the court procedure under paragraph 9 of the same Law (JGG 1988); the judge may also decide on a community service order or probation as a prerequisite for the suspension of the court procedure.

THE PILOT PROJECT

In May 1987 a pilot project, the *Ausserstrafrechtliche Konfliktregelung im Jugendgerichtsverfahren* (Out of Court Conflict Resolution in Juvenile Justice Matters) was completed, a final report was drawn up and on 16 June 1987 its results were presented by the Minister of Justice as an important piece of reform to be incorporated in the proposed juvenile justice legislation. The new Juvenile Justice Law came into force on 1 January 1989. This kind of description of events does not attempt to exaggerate the role which was played by the pilot project and the way in which it influenced criminal law. However, in Austria we are now talking not only about dealing with young offenders but also about adult criminal law in general; the pilot project has had some significance for this development.

In order to understand what happened in the pilot project more thoroughly, I want to present some theoretical thinking about alternatives to criminal law concepts as well as a description of the project itself – that is the implementation of this kind of theoretical thinking. My intention is to give at least a general outline and a sketch of the very complex process, involving intertwining political forces, interests and expectations, that determines both the making and the outcome of an experiment in criminal justice in a small country.

But to add flesh and life to the theoretical skeleton and to the bones of analysis, I want to start with a few stories from the Austrian

Juvenile Court and from within the experiment in conflict resolution.

Examples of cases in Austrian Juvenile Court

First, in a Viennese youth club, several youngsters had made a nuisance of themselves. The director threw them out, including one who had not been really involved, who insisted on either being allowed to stay or getting back his entrance fee. The leader kept to his decision to order him out and to forbid further visits. In this situation the boy resorted to a kind of self-help. He uttered a threat toward the director (which could be loosely translated as 'I'll clobber you'), took several packages of ice-cream out of the refrigerator (which were of equivalent value to the entrance fee) and made his way out. The director reported the event to the police and the youth was charged with *räuberische Erpressung* (blackmailing by means of robbery) which is an offence defined thus:

> Whoever is pressing somebody by means of force or dangerous threat to do something, let something be done or leave something that results in a damage to somebody else's property, is to be punished with confinement from six months to five years if he has acted with the intention of illegally enriching himself or a third person.
>
> (paragraph 144 of the *Österreichisches Strafgesetzbuch* [Austrian Book of Penal law]: commonly abbreviated to 144 *StGB*)

Second, a 17-year-old youngster had served a conditional sentence because of theft and minor bodily injury in a youth reformatory (which was closed in 1974). After his release, he shared a flat with his girlfriend who, after a while, wanted a separation. He tried to fight her decision and the girl, feeling rather helpless, reported to the police that she had been verbally threatened and intimidated by her boyfriend. In the course of formal investigations the charge proved void of content. However, while in his apartment, the youngster was hauled off by the police. He resisted and there was some scuffling with the officers. The police report alleged that the young man had bitten the calf of an officer, had hit and scratched him. He was charged with *Körperverletzung* (bodily assault) under paragraph 83 *StGB*, which states 'Whoever impedes a public agency or a civil servant in the execution of an official duty, and is thereby using force or threatens to use force is to be punished with confinement of up to six months or with a fine up to 360 "day-units" ' and with *Widerstand gegen die Staatsgewalt* (resistance to public order) under paragraph 269 *StGB*, which states 'Whoever hinders a state institution or a civil servant, by force or by threatening to use force, hinders in the execution of an official act, is to be punished with confinement up to three years.' These charges resulted in a five-month prison sentence which was to be imposed immediately because of his previous conviction.

Examples of cases of conflict resolution

The following three stories of conflict resolution present a clear contrast with the stories from the Juvenile Court.

First, a youngster had been caught by the police while driving a motor vehicle without the owner's consent, having broken the lock by force. The vehicle had been returned to its owner. The social worker handling the case inside the project contacted the young man and asked him to give a detailed account of the event. Then he wrote a letter to the victim asking him to arrange a date to talk about this demands concerning material compensation. In this conversation, the young offender, the victim and the social worker took part. The rooms of the local probation office served as a meeting-place. The owner of the vehicle used the opportunity to talk sense with the youngster, to tell him in no uncertain terms about his rage on finding that his vehicle had been stolen and about the nuisance he had experienced while trying to recover it. When the question of compensation and of paying for the damaged lock at last popped up, he waved it off, saying 'Keep your money, you are more in need of it than I am.' The state prosecutor dropped the charge.

Second, in the countryside in the province of Upper Austria, a group of young people had, for quite a while, been amusing themselves by interfering with and breaking open gambling machines. In addition they had committed a series of minor burglaries and had damaged motor vehicles. The state prosecutor supplied the social worker with a long list of the offences brought to the notice of the police and with the names of the offenders and their victims. Two of the project's social workers visited the village and spoke with the considerable number of its residents who had been affected by the goings-on. They talked to the youngsters, to their families, some of whom appeared very upset about their sons' exploits, and to the innkeepers who had been the victims of much of the delinquent activity. All of them proved very understanding, helpful and co-operative. Agreements as to the compensation to be paid were made and in quite a few of the cases the amount fixed was below that originally stated in the police files. Several offenders were over 18 and were therefore not subject to Juvenile Justice Law regulations. Nevertheless they joined the venture and participated in the compensation payments. In most of the cases concerning the juveniles, preconditions sufficient to dismiss the charge by the state prosecutor could be procured. Young adult offenders got away with a mitigated sentence.

Third, in the *Prater* (a kind of amusement park in Vienna) two young men on their way back from some excessively 'moistened' merriment took a motor vehicle to carry them home. The vehicle broke down and the police caught the youngsters while they were pushing it along. Its owner, a young Pakistani newspaper-seller (a dangerous and low-paid job selling newspapers on the roadside) was aggrieved by the loss of the vehicle, which was essential for his job. The social worker got in contact first with the two young men, and afterwards with the victim, who in the beginning proved rather reluctant, even defensive, to talk about ways of arranging compensation. On the other hand, the boys voiced their opinion that the vehicle had been in a very poor condition anyway and compensation payments ought to be reduced accordingly. When the 'big talk', at which the social worker also was present, at last took place, it was heated and intense. The offenders appeared disconcerted and deeply impressed by the dreary picture which the newspaper-seller drew of the circumstances of his life and work. An agreement about compensation payments was reached, being a compromise between the victim's first demand and the offenders' first offer; it was to be paid in three instalments. The state prosecutor dropped the indictment.

The overall picture of conflict resolution in juvenile justice matters in Austria is, as I have hinted, neither straightforward nor simple. It is marked by three contradictions or paradoxes. First, there is the contradiction between the clear-cut and radical social policy concept of the 're-appropriation of conflicts' which underlay the project, on the one hand, and the rather more pragmatic, workable design for making the project run, on the other. Second, we find the paradoxical fact that, what is entitled 'out of court' conflict resolution, was in fact based in the State Prosecutor's Office, implying that the very agency that represents the monopoly of power by the state (*staatliches Gewaltmonopol*) is entrusted with the task of repressing state-induced repression. Third, and finally, there is a contradiction within the design of research that went with the project in so far as it was at the same time both action research and evaluation research. The *Institut für Rechts-und Kriminalsoziologie* (Institute of the Sociology of Law and Crime) provided objective data on the workings of the pilot project and at the same time took part in the ongoing policy-making process by reporting and discussing data and observations with the people involved. This was termed *Begleitforschung* (accompanying research). Although *The Statistics of the Success of the Conflict Resolution Scheme* (Pelikan and Pilgram 1988; 55–79) served as an important piece of argument in policy discussions, it did not, in our opinion, account for the considerable political success of the experiment in the first place. Policy-making proved to be an ongoing process, a mutual exchange between the experience derived from practice, politics and theoretical thinking. Science and research became actors on the stage of conscientious policy-making.

THEORETICAL CONCEPTS AND EMPIRICAL DATA

The concept of the 're-appropriation of conflicts' that served as a basis for our work is an alternative to the conventions of criminal law in two ways. First, it implies a different perception and second a different handling of events that become relevant within the framework of the criminal law. The kind of everyday-reasoning on which this concept is built runs thus: delinquent acts ought to be perceived as social conflicts, as damages, as torts, as encroachments on somebody's rights, as a nuisance or a disturbance that happened to somebody. Very many of these conflicts are dealt with in one way or another between the opponents, by communicating, by quarrelling, by just letting the matter drop, by talking to others or by enlisting mental and/or physical help of a third party. It is therefore only a small portion of these conflicts that is reported to the police and therefore comes to the notice of the state prosecutor. At that point what has been termed the 'expropriation of conflicts' takes place, meaning that the event is defined and handled according to the logic of the criminal code and no longer according to the needs and interests of the parties involved.

The assets of criminal law as the most advanced institution of 'formal social control' include impartiality, objectivity and equality. But these assets are counterbalanced by a liability, namely the stark inability of positive criminal law to restore the social equilibrium or balance that has been disturbed by an event which has been defined as criminal. In other words, it is not capable of effecting immediate social integration. A scheme of conflict resolution can be seen as an attempt to overcome this deficiency by re-establishing elements and procedures of informal social control and at the same time preserving the main assets of the formal institutions.

During the last five years much empirical research data, quantitative as well as qualitative, has been brought together by members of the Institute of the Sociology of Law and the Sociology of Deviance in Vienna, partly in co-operation with researchers in the same field at Frankfurt University. The most recent of this research pertains to the perception and to the handling of conflicts in everyday life. On the basis of the data assembled, 1,100 'conflict stories' were collected, recorded and submitted to qualitative analysis and an ethnography of conflicts was created (Hanak *et al.* 1989). A very rough outline of these findings indicates that sanctioning the opponent is a strategy used in only 15 per cent of the conflict-stories gathered. Included are informal sanctions such as the use of physical violence as well as reactions of 'demonstrative avoidance' on the one hand and formal sanctions (the mobilisation of the agencies of formal control) on the other. The latter accounts for no more than 5 per cent of all cases and among those the stories ending up with a criminal indictment constitute the tiny minority of just 1 per cent. The vast majority of everyday conflicts are handled in a way that has been labelled 'absorption of conflicts' (Hanak 1987: 29). Partly this is achieved by belittling the kind of nuisance that has been caused by only a minor disturbance which can be easily corrected – by trifling with a trifle, one could say. Or people might just get resigned to the tort or damage which has been inflicted upon them; this happens often after some time has elapsed, time having not only healed wounds but also permitted material losses to be made good. This also happens when the injured party has material or non-material resources to overcome the loss or grievance experienced.

There remains a type of conflict which can be handled by

communicating about it, either with or without the help of an intermediary. Conflicts arising out of formal or informal claims, or cases that have to do with wilful destruction, are appropriate for this sort of solution. A willingness to co-operate is prerequisite for both parties and additionally a certain amount of knowledge, experience, and of confidence on the part of the aggrieved party is needed for them to take the initiative. This is of course the constellation where the agencies of civil law as well as institutions specialising in the defence and enforcement of claims might step in, making a contribution toward conflict resolution. This is also one of the main fields for out-of-court conflict resolution, as was attempted in our project.

Although these results are well established, I would not dare to extrapolate them to another western European society, let alone a Common Law country such as Great Britain. Nevertheless this attempt to establish an 'ethnography of dealing with conflicts', together with the inadequacy of the agencies of formal control, point to something that might hold true in any of the societies which we label *rechtsstaatlich* (a state ordered by law and adhering to law), irrespective of whether it is characterised by Common Law or Roman Law. They serve to underline the rather trivial fact that the law, and particularly criminal law, plays a rather insignificant role in the everyday life of ordinary people. This should not be taken as an invitation just to throw one's hands up in resignation but rather to think constructively about those alternatives that are located outside formal criminal procedure.

What we have stated theoretically as the overall aim of conflict resolution – the re-establishment of elements and procedures of informal social control – can now be translated into practice. If we succeed in 'giving back the conflict', offering a re-appropriation of the conflict, asking the injured party to express what kind of compensation or reparation he or she wants from the person that has done him or her some harm, or caused damage, we serve the victim's interest better than by setting up a trial and we also spare the young offender the stigma of a criminal record. Under these circumstances, the state prosecutor should take the reparation or reconciliation agreed upon by both parties as sufficient proof that further intervention has become unnecessary and that the public has no further interest in the prosecution. He can drop the indictment.

AN EXPERIMENT WITHIN THE JUDICIAL SYSTEM

One of the last initiatives of the great reform era under the Minister of Justice, Christian Broda, was a first draft for the new Juvenile Justice Law in 1982. It introduced a diversion programme offering the instrument of Community Service Orders which followed the example of the *Brücke* Project in Munich. Work instead of punishment (the 'utopia of regenerative toil', as Faugeron and Houchon (1987) had called it; work in social service institutions, in homes for elderly people, in institutions for handicapped children and, work in hospitals) was an idea, which was greeted with considerable enthusiasm by representatives of the judiciary. It was not stated in print, but it was understood, that the Austrian Probation Service and Social Work Association should organise and supervise these Community Service Orders. But this reform idea met with considerable scepticism and opposition. This scheme was against the self-image and against the criminal policy intentions of the Probation Service Association. To execute orders of the court and to be used as an agency of control – in the narrow sense of social control – seemed intolerable. So the call for an alternative to the alternative was heard.

It coincided with a growing tendency within the Austrian State Prosecutor's Office to dismiss charges when dealing with minor juvenile offences. Again I have to extemporise. There is a paragraph within the then existing Austrian Juvenile Justice Law stating that the prosecutor can renounce, or – more figuratively – step back from, the prosecution (*Absehen von der Strafverfolgung*) whenever he expects or presumes that in case of an indictment the defendant would be sentenced to no more than a small fine or a short term of imprisonment, notwithstanding considerations of special deterrence.

Thus on tiptoes the *Opportunitätsprinzip* (principle of discretion) seems at last to have entered Austrian criminal procedural law and, most interesting, in a way that is likely to strengthen the authority of the State Prosecutor's office. The use of his right to drop an indictment is interpreted as 'negative sentencing' or 'negative justice'; the prosecutor is still the 'master of the criminal procedure'. Anyway, this newly opened realm of negative justice could be used to provide the prosecutor with a kind of information or reasoning on which to base his anticipation of a lenient sentence.

In anticipating the judge's sentence, the prosecutor should, according to the *Kommentare* (the handbook based on the Law Codes which provides guidelines for judges and lawyers), concentrate his or her attention on the probability of a favourable prognosis for the youth's career, favourable in the sense that no criminal career is to be expected. Could not the consideration of a dismissal of the charge be extended by basing this prognosis on the fact that crucial events, such as reparation and reconciliation, had taken place since the delinquent act had happened and that reparation and reconciliation had taken place? Could not such goings-on be taken as a sign, an indicator, that things might turn out to be all right, because they had already been set on the right path?

Up to this point, I have been arguing from the point of view of the judiciary, who needed to find an opening, some margin, in the existing law which could be used to legitimise an experiment. One has to keep in mind that the mere idea of an experiment within the criminal law system is in opposition to the concept of continental positive law and to the principle of equality before the law. So there was strong opposition within the State Prosecutor's Office. This opposition has now been overcome by the sheer success of the pilot project. But as already mentioned, it was the Austrian Probation Service and Social Work Association that had put forward the idea of an experiment as a means to express and to advocate its criminal policy intentions. The theoretical foundations as well as the design for 'accompanying research' were outlined by the Institute of the Sociology of Law and the Sociology of Crime which had from its creation maintained close personal and ideological relations to the Association. This fact helps to explain the way in which this kind of research was set up and accomplished.

THE PRACTICE AND THE PROBLEMS OF OUT OF COURT CONFLICT RESOLUTION IN AUSTRIA

The experiment started in Linz in spring 1985 and in Vienna and Salzburg in September 1985. The ideal-type reparation scheme I have outlined above describes the main content and the overall aim of the pilot project. But we took a rather pragmatic line of action. The idea was to try out a range of alternative measures, to establish trust in the working of such alternatives and to facilitate comparison between different modes of social intervention. For example, there was a part of the programme located at the court (not at the Prosecutors' office) at the magistrate's level, as well as at the superior court, dealing with juvenile delinquency in Salzburg. In those cases, the outcome of conflict resolution was used in the course of the court proceedings and resulted in mitigation of sentence, at best in the admonition (*Ermahnung*) of the offender by the judge.

There existed different modes of co-operation and communication between the prosecutor or the judge and the social workers. These modes of co-operation are in a way dependent on the allocation of discretionary powers as concerns the selection of cases for conflict resolution. In the first place it was the prosecutor, or a 'team' of prosecutors, who decided which cases ought to go all the way back to where they started from – the conflict between the victim and the offender. Social workers participated to varying degrees in this process. In Salzburg the social worker together with the judge at magistrate's level went through all the files of a certain period of time and took out those where a kind of conflict resolution seemed feasible as well as potentially beneficial for the parties involved.

In Linz, social workers attended the regular sessions of the state prosecutors, where they were confronted with the cases the prosecutors considered 'suitable' for reparation and reconciliation. They were asked their opinion as to suitability and as to the methods they would apply. A kind of inter-professional talk and communication took place.

In Vienna, the domain of competence of the prosecutor and the social worker remained strictly separated. The prosecutors chose the cases and informed the social workers of their decision. The social workers in return informed the prosecutors of the result of the intervention and that formed the basis of the prosecutor's decision to renounce the charge or to prosecute.

Nevertheless in trying to depict the overall development within the project one might very rightly talk of a 'triumph of the State Prosecutors'. They succeeded not only in keeping, but also in extending their role of gatekeeper in criminal justice procedures. Thus within the 'Austrian model' of conflict resolution it is the state prosecutors who exercise discretion as to whether a case that has come to their notice is to be handed back to the people out of whose conflicts it has arisen or whether an indictment is drawn up.

It is up to them to renounce further state intervention according to the penal code if they regard the results of an informal agreement brought about by the intervention and the help of the social worker as 'sufficient'. This paradox of enlarging the discretionary powers of the state agency cannot be denied, but it can be explained out of the history and existing structures of this institution. Briefly, the conflict resolution scheme had offered state prosecutors a real chance to rebuild and redefine their role, which had involved their being able to concentrate on people instead of files. Close contact and co-operation with social workers of the pilot project encouraged this change but it had already begun to happen when the experiment started. This took the shape of the prosecutor trying to use conflict resolution as a way of educating young people, and their trying to use it as a way of diagnosing social and even psychic needs which they thought called for some kind of intervention.

At this point we encounter the sensitive topic of the net-widening effect contained in and promoted by the project. It was there both as a danger and as a problem. The educational aspirations of prosecutors – catching up at last with the judges in the field of juvenile justice – were and are apt to blur the very policy intentions of the conflict resolution scheme which were, and I emphasise, the renunciation of any kind of state intervention – of both the repressive and punishing and the correcting and educational kinds.

As a matter of fact, this kind of problem, the danger of net-widening, or of (mis)understanding and (ab)using conflict resolution as just another diversion programme is not only inherent in the thinking and in the aspirations of the judiciary but also can be traced to the diversity the experiment offered in handling the cases. As was mentioned above, a wide range of offences were included in the programme and correspondingly a wide range of instruments for dealing with cases applied. Especially during the first months of the experiment we even resorted to a kind of Community Service Order although now these cases are exceptional. But we have kept up the practice of offering young people who got involved in a traffic offence, at least those which indicated a more deeply rooted problem in handling vehicles and/or traffic situations, a very individually designed course consisting of one or several sessions. Also the Probation Service and Social Work Association uses its contacts with a wide range of social assistance organisations for procuring special help for special needs that become visible during the conflict resolution procedure. But we have stressed the fact that any kind of 'treatment' the offender undergoes in one of those organisations must not be brought to bear on the assessment and the 'judgement' of the procedure of conflict resolution and its outcome. The state prosecutor has to rely exclusively on the kind of settlement and the kind of compensation agreed upon, on the restoration of social balance and of a status quo that is acceptable to the parties.

SCHEMES OF CONFLICT RESOLUTION IN THE FRG – THE PRECONDITIONS

When talking of conflict resolution in the FRG one has again to start by providing some background information, first about the characteristics of the penal process. In recent years there have been considerable efforts to strengthen the position of the victim within criminal law procedures. This was to be effected by various means; besides private prosecution there exists *Nebenklage* ('supplementary prosecution') and the application for a judicial decision against a public prosecutor's decision to renounce indictment. In addition a follow-up procedure for civil claims was enacted – similar to the *action civile en reparation du dommage* of the French penal procedure. An assessment of the impact and the factual use made of these legal provisions stated that this system lacks 'the necessary clarity, cohesion and practicability to be effective for the victim' (Villmow 1984: 17). According to a report on victim compensation drawn up quite recently by the *Bundesverband der Straffälligenhilfe* (Association for Assistance to Offenders) this is explained partly by the fact that the traditionally rigid separation of penal and civil procedures within the respective German law codes makes for a kind of mental barrier against widespread and 'fluent' use of the *action civile* in the FRG (Bundesministerium der Justiz 1988: 26).

Another important enhancement of the position of the victim was provided by Juvenile Criminal Law containing a *Wiedergutmachungsauflage* (compensation order). The German Juvenile Justice Law has been in force since 1923. A lengthy debate had preceded its enactment. It had concentrated upon the significance and the efficacy of the principle of legality (*Legalitätsprinzip*) as related to juvenile justice. A set-back or a partial infringement of its dominating influence aimed at opening up better opportunities for educational intervention and 'treatment' was advocated by representatives of the 'Modern Penal Law School'. The compensation order can be seen within the context of state-imposed 'rehabilitative' measures. It serves as a precondition for the dismissal of the charge by the state prosecutor under paragraph 45 of the German *Jugendgerichtgesetz* (45 *JGG*) as well as for a suspension of procedure (*Verfahrenseinstellung*) by the judge under 47 *JGG*. Though wider use is made of these possibilities than of similar provisions within the Penal Code for adults they are not used as a means of involving victim and offender in a process of reparation and an attempt for reconciliation.

On the other hand the situation in the field of juvenile justice in the FRG has been marked by the thriving of various diversion programmes during the last decade, the *Brücke* programme in Munich being the largest and most well known. These projects once again were motivated by the need to find something more sensible and more effective than confinement or the threat of confinement; once more the 'utopia of regenerative toil' (Faugeron and Houchon 1987: 400) was evoked. But only a little later disillusionment spread and criticism of the rehabilitative ideals and of treatment in general became more pronounced. It coincided with efforts to provide more effectively for victims' needs and interests and generated a wide range of conflict resolution programmes all over the FRG. Nevertheless one might rightly discriminate between victim-oriented, offender-oriented projects and conflict resolution schemes proper. The modes of organisation and of financing also varies considerably. Projects are organised partly by *freie Träger* (independent welfare organisations), partly by municipalities, and partly by the judiciary; there are also combinations of state, municipal, and private/independent agencies.

I shall select only three of the programmes to present an outline of their policy intentions and their content.

The *Waage-Projekt* in Cologne was founded in 1986 by an association established especially for the purpose. Financial support is provided by a private foundation and by a state programme. There exists an 'accompanying research' programme, which is carried out within the project itself (*Jahresbericht die Waage* 1987; Bundesministerium der Justiz 1988: 18).

The goal stated by its supporters is to try out modes of victim–offender mediation involving juvenile as well as young adult offenders and hence to establish conflict resolution schemes within the jurisdiction of the *Amtsgericht* (magistrates' court) in Cologne. Selection of cases to be handled within the project is done either by the state prosecutor or by the judge. The project worker contacts the young offenders to ascertain their readiness to participate and then visits the victims to find out about their expectations as to consequences of the offence and about their willingness to co-operate. The process of mediation itself is attempted with the help of a third person functioning as a mediator. The agreement arrived at and its fulfilment is brought to the notice of the state prosecutor or the judge and is used as basis for 'concluding' the procedure, that is by either dropping the indictment or by suspending the procedure.

About 230 young offenders and their victims had been in the project by the beginning of 1989 (Schreckling 1989). The kinds of offences handled within the mediation scheme should be in the middle-range of 'seriousness', which means that even repeated robbery and assault could be included. In the course of the project the most common offences dealt with have been acts of violence against the person. As in Austria, the willingness of both offenders and victims to co-operate in the mediation scheme was extremely high (90–95 per cent). The same holds true for the rate of settlements agreed upon and also for the rate of their reaching a successful conclusion. Reparation often included financial compensation by the young offenders to their victims. There is one last result stressed by the preliminary report – namely that the meeting of the parties involved in the event is often an important opportunity to come to terms with what has happened. This means that the offender is confronted with the consequences of inflicting pain on somebody and the meeting also permits the victim to express fear and anger. Because of the strength of feeling which may be involved, careful preparation and a high degree of professional competence and of continuing reflection by the social worker as a mediator must be assured.

The *Braunschweiger Modellversuch* is located at the *Jugendgerichtshilfe* (Juvenile Court Assistance Association) in Braunschweig and is supported by a foundation (the *Deutsche Jugendmarke e.V.*) as well as by the Ministry of Justice of Niedersachsen. Evaluation research is being carried out by the *Kriminologisches Forschungsinstitut*

Niedersachsen e.V. (Criminological Research Institute of Lower Saxony) (Bundesministerium der Justiz 1988: 18; Schmitz and Hassebrauck 1987).

As far as its policy intentions are concerned, the project subscribes to the theory of re-appropriation of conflicts, although specific goals are defined for different fields of action. There is an educational object to be effected in relation to the offender – by the process of mediation itself; an institutional effect is also intended by reducing the caseload processed by the courts. Furthermore the victim is to be thought of: providing the opportunity to reduce fear and prejudice against young people in general is stated as an explicit aim of the project.

In the *Braunschweiger Modell* only individual not institutional victims are included, meaning that traffic offences or shoplifting are not dealt with. Another prerequisite is the undisputed confession of the offender. One of the special features of the *Braunschweiger Modell* is the attempt to start conflict resolution at a very early point, before an indictment is drawn up by the state prosecutor or even immediately after a case has been reported to the police. Therefore co-operation of the Braunschweig police was sought, though results about the success of this aspect of the programme will need some more time before they can be evaluated; at a workshop in Bonn in June 1989 (see below) participants were told that – after some difficulties in the beginning – police co-operation proved fruitful (Viet 1989).

As concerns the mediation process itself, emphasis is laid upon the discourse between victim and offender, their talking together preferably in the presence of the social worker of the Juvenile Court Assistance Association.

The preliminary results of the Braunschweig project show comparatively low participation rates of offenders as well as of victims. One might suspect that the highly official character of the Juvenile Court Assistance Association and the fact that it is perceived as a part of the court is responsible for some reluctance on the side of the parties to be contacted. In addition there is some indication that the social workers of the Juvenile Court Assistance Association might have encountered considerable difficulties in adapting to their new role as mediators.

The *Projekt Handschlag* in Reutlingen (in Baden-Württemberg) focuses on the 'big talk', the discourse between offender and victim, ending up in the symbolic gesture of the joining of hands. It is organised by a private association together with the Institute for Educational Sciences at the University of Tübingen, in close co-operation with the Juvenile Court Assistance Association and the judiciary. Financial support is provided by the Baden-Württemberg Ministry for the Family, Youth and Health (Bundesministerium der Justiz 1988: 20; Kuhn 1987).

This project also concentrates on personal (as distinct from anonymous or corporate) victims and there must also be a confession of guilt by the offender. Minor offences are explicitly excluded.

Different instruments are applied for bringing about reparation. There can be joint work by both parties to make repairs for the damage done. In some cases, especially when the offence was assault, a 'joint venture', aimed at some kind of community service, could be initiated, such as cleaning up a local brook. Financial reparation to the victim can also be made out of a special fund, supplied by payments for services provided by offenders. Finally presents may be given to the victim which are understood to be symbolic gestures of reconciliation.

The criminal policy intentions that lie behind the application of these instruments could be characterised as stimulating and helping both parties in their attempt to arrive at a working compromise for the conflict they have experienced. Annette Kuhn and Dieter Rössner (1987) who designed the project have pointed to the integrative potential of conflict resolution procedures as opposed to the primary function of institutions of formal control which is to make clear and to stress norms (*Normverdeutlichung*). It is obvious that the *Projekt Handschlag* is very similar to the Austrian conflict resolution scheme, although there is a somewhat heavier emphasis laid upon the educational effects of the mediation effort – at least in theory. The project in Reutlingen is a very well-designed programme and is well grounded in *Sozialpädagogik* (educational theory), although it is a rather small-scale programme as far as the number of cases is concerned; fewer than one hundred were completed within one year.

Results of the research done on *Projekt Handschlag* have shown that a high proportion of both victims and young offenders are prepared to be involved in the mediation effort. Again experience of motives and expectations of victims about prosecution and the 'criminalisation' of offenders coincide to a large extent with the kinds of results obtained in the pilot project in Austria (Pelikan 1987: 91–110).

Meanwhile conflict resolution has gained nation-wide recognition in the FRG and its formal incorporation in Juvenile Justice Legislation is being considered. In June 1989 the German Probation Service Association organised an intensive workshop on the results of various conflict resolution schemes. During the final discussion on their future and their impact on criminal policy in general the Minister of Justice, Hans Engelhardt, and President Richard von Weizsäcker were present. Agreement was reached as concerns the necessity of continuing experimental projects, of further assessment of their results and of their being accepted by victims and offenders. But opinions vary about the appropriate organisation framework for establishing conflict resolution on a large scale. The Juvenile Court Assistance Association, the Probation Service Association, the police and independent welfare organisations each offer competing arguments for their own potential to deal with the new social task. However, the situation was resolved by the consensus that legal provisions at this stage were regarded as premature; more planning, research, and political work was to be done first.

The Austrian model of conflict resolution and the Austrian legislation in the field of juvenile justice has exercised considerable influence on policy-makers in the FRG. Of even greater importance proved to be the setting up of a working group of Austrian and German practitioners and researchers involved in the field of conflict resolution. Based on their collective experience, they succeeded, in the summer of 1989, in drawing up guidelines and standards for professional work in this new field. They have endeavoured to establish a kind of internal 'communicative' control as a safeguard against the loss of professional quality but even more importantly as a means of preserving and developing further the overall social policy goal of conflict resolution. There is a certain danger that the programme might deteriorate and become something like 'a crash course in probation by enforced reparation and repentence involving the victim' (Werdenich 1988: 135). Only careful training of social workers and continuous control by communicating and by reflecting upon the process of conflict resolution can prevent this development actually taking place.

The lesson of the Austrian experience and of co-operation within mediation projects in the FRG is this: conflict resolution is not just a procedure to prevent an offender's further progress on a criminal career. Conflict resolution means using, encouraging and strengthening the capacity of people to deal with the material and emotional damages and grievances that have been created by the intentional and unintentional deeds of people or groups of people against the integrity and the interests of their fellow human-beings; it means that one learns to trust in this potential and to enlist the help and the services necessary to support and restore this capacity, whenever they prove deficient. This calls for a clear perspective, careful planning and even more careful implementation of conflict resolution programmes. A delicate balance of intervention and restraint has to be achieved, when handing back the conflicts to be handled according to the needs and interests of the people involved. Conflict resolution is not a panacea for the ills of society and for the wrong-doings which people experience. It is a small step within a small area of everyday life towards more personal autonomy, and greater control of one's own life.

©1991 Christa Pelikan

Chapter twelve

Developments in business crime control in Europe

Michael Levi

INTRODUCTION

Despite the use made of 'white-collar crime' by Sutherland (1983, first published 1939) to attack biological or poverty-based theories of crime, the incorporation into criminology of crimes by and against business remains at best fitful. Commercial crime is absent from almost all the recent interest in 'The Victim' (Fattah 1986), including victimisation *surveys* which – even in the rare cases where crime risks at work are examined (Mayhew *et al.* 1989: ch. 4) – are devoted principally to natural persons suffering at the hands of other natural persons or groups, and which thereby unintentionally reinforce popular ideologies of what 'crime' constitutes and who 'the criminals' and 'the victims' are. International crime and policing – of which white-collar crime is a sub-set – are even more neglected, with no real follow-up to the pioneering work of Mack (1975) on 'the crime industry': Anderson (1989) devotes almost no attention to fraud, counterfeiting, or any other property asportation crimes in his discussion of the politics of international police co-operation, and this in turn largely reflects the greater police interest in cross-border drug-trafficking and terrorism than in theft and deception.

Looking at multinational – as contrasted with international – studies of crime, despite the plea of the Council of Europe (1981) for detailed collation of data on economic crime, it is very rare for fraud to receive any attention in most countries' annual reports on the costs of crime. The Dutch Social and Cultural Planning Report (1986: 206) observes that tax evasion was three times greater than the combined total of private and public sector crime costs, though this is complicated by the fact that embezzlement and shoplifting estimates ranged widely from 20 million to 1,000 million guilders: but even this relative sophistication excludes health and safety, cartels, and environmental offences, whose financial or even human impact is more difficult to estimate. This is also the case with the interesting Home Office (1988b) *Report of the Working Group on the Costs of Crime.* Fraud and other forms of business crime are neglected even in European discussions of crime *prevention*: see, for example, the valuable *Special European Edition of the Home Office Research Bulletin* (1987). Consequently it is unsurprising that hard data – even official data – about business crime and its control in European countries are unavailable, and this will be reflected in the patchwork discussion in this article.

The title of this article begs a number of questions that have no self-evident solutions. First, what is meant by Europe? Do we mean the European Community (EC) or something wider, including – in these days of *perestroika* – 'Eastern' European countries whose economic systems are no longer so dissimilar from those of the west? Second, what do we mean by 'in' Europe? Should we include frauds by European businesses against those wholly outside Europe? Do we mean frauds against European victims, no matter whether plotted and executed from Europe or outside it? (What if only part was conceived in Europe?) In this connection, it is of interest that firms outside as well as inside the European Community (EC) can be fined for making (or implementing) agreements which substantially prevent, restrict or distort competition in the Common Market. Third, what do we mean by 'business crime?' Do we wish to include not only fraud *by* the use of corporations but also fraud (such as credit card fraud) *against* corporations by private individuals? Do we include conduct that has *not* led to any conviction in any court (1) with criminal jurisdiction or (2) with administrative jurisdiction that imposes penalties upon those adjudicated as guilty? Should we include not only fraud but also health and safety offences, pollution, anti-competitive practices, and so on, which is what many criminologists (see Braithwaite 1984 in his study of the pharmaceutical industry) would mean by the term 'corporate crime'? How would we construe, for example, the relevance to this topic of Italian companies dumping toxic waste in parts of West Africa where, at the time – 1988/89 – this was not illegal, or even where anti-dumping laws were evaded by the bribery of public officials in Africa (i.e. outside Europe)? Or to allegations in the European and Indian press that Swedish armaments manufacturers bribed Indian defence contractors and possibly leading politicians in the Rajiv Ghandi government to give them orders for goods, perhaps laundering their deals through British companies, with or without the knowledge of the latter that the deals were artificial? These examples illustrate the problems that the EC, let alone individual nation-states, has in combating business crime. (They also raise problems for the conventional wisdom of ecologists of crime that 'crime' is predominantly local in character.) Given the space available here, I will focus principally on control in Britain, though other European countries are examined briefly here and in collections elsewhere (see, for edited work in English, Leigh 1980; Magnusson 1985; Leigh and Smith, forthcoming).

SHIFTS IN FINANCIAL CRIME CONTROL IN EUROPE

For present purposes, I shall take national legislation and official control agencies as the context for discussion, since although much fraud and corporate 'regulatory violations' may have become international in character, efforts to control them are still predominantly based on notions of national sovereignty (Anderson 1989). Unless our conception of 'crime' is purely subjective or we have some conceptual warrant for standardising discussion – as advocated by Wilkins (1984) who suggests that comparative analysts should not discuss 'crime' but 'social harms' which are less subject to legislative vagaries – the definition of business *crime* depends upon legislation and upon the law-in-action. It is here that we encounter the first serious difficulties: even within the EC, each country has different substantive legislation, police powers, and policing levels and strategies. In this sense, one may write of European *countries*' methods of dealing with corporate crime, but less plausibly of European control *per se*, except in very specific areas where the ministerial-level TREVI group discusses public order control in Europe or the European Commission's supranational responsibility runs parallel to (or in conflict with) national legislation. Legislation affecting cross-border activities creates many problems of comity between jurisdictions (*Law and Contemporary Problems* 1987; Levi, forthcoming), and it should be appreciated that instead of explaining the regulation of corporate crime as a static phenomenon, one must examine and account for its dynamics over time. In addition to any national and international developments in the control of insider trading, narcotics, banking fraud, and terrorism (Levi, forthcoming), there are specific features of control that emanate from Europe via the responsibility of the European Commission for banking and securities regulation, company law, and competition policy (Steiner 1988). In trying to describe and account for these dynamics, I shall use my own interview sources as well as documentary material.

Exchanges of information between other European states are much smoother than such exchanges between the UK and the rest of Europe. There is one simple reason for this: whereas civil law countries working on written Penal Codes – i.e. all of the EC except the UK – are able to supply cross-border information readily via letters of request or *commissions rogatoires*, the UK does not recognise European examining magistrates as competent *judicial* authorities for the supply of information in criminal proceedings, since they are investigators, not (in UK eyes) independent judges. Ironically, in the light of generally more lenient attitudes towards tax evasion than against other frauds in respect of bank secrecy, the cross-border problem may be *less* in tax matters, since the OECD (1989) – which represents major economic powers inside and outside the EC – proposes an unprecedented level of information sharing between member states (with the ability to restrict it on occasions). The 1989 OECD Convention expressly states, however, that such taxation information-sharing agreements do not override any rules made by the EC to govern member activities.

The problem of international co-operation is not, however, a purely legal problem: it is also a problem of culture – attitudes and language – and of interests. Particularly when pressures for organisational performance have built-in indicators, matters considered (or, just as often, *not* considered at all) to be extraneous to the goals of the organisation are given a low priority, and except when given explicit high-profile interest, international frauds that do no direct harm to the country where the police and prosecutors are stationed are not prime candidates for attention. (Except in global businesses like securities trading, the effects of fraud upon the long-term commercial reputation of the country is not a real consideration in practice). Indeed, at one stage in the 1980s, the English Director of Public Prosecutions had a general policy of not prosecuting frauds committed from English territory where there were no victims in the UK (Levi 1987a). Although such policies no longer exist at a formal level, they are part of the informal taken-for-granted assumptions built into policing priorities, except where overturned specifically by orders from senior police, sometimes influenced by the media and politicians. When this inertia as regards cases with no local victims is overcome, it is normally as a result of the informal police culture of social networks developed by meeting (and drinking) at conferences, courses, or on attachment to Interpol. Let us now examine European control trends in some specific areas.

Securities frauds

As in other spheres of crime control, the control of securities frauds in Europe has been nation-based, though international meetings of securities regulators – like banking regulators – are now held, and these are supplemented by frequent informal and formal communications. As regards the UK, it is important to realise the effects of two major trends: first, the Financial Services Act 1986 (now in force) requires the UK Securities and Investments Board (SIB) to be satisfied by the fitness *and* the propriety of any corporate or individual person selling securities to investors in the UK. There are no completely satisfactory definitions of what being fit and proper means, though it involves at least not having a criminal record for 'serious' theft or fraud, and demonstrating some minimal competence and financial resources. However, given the internationalisation of the securities *industry*, the fit and proper person requirement creates problems because of disparities in regulatory standards within EC and other European countries. Matters that are unlawful in the UK are permitted, say, in Italy both at a formal legal level and at a practical, enforcement one, with higher rates of monitoring of securities conduct in the UK than elsewhere. This causes 'downstream' problems of international enforcement, because if we rely upon formal adjudications of misconduct as the basis for prohibiting people from engaging in securities trading we understate the potential violators from countries that have lax formal regulation; whereas if we go beyond this and rely on market rumour, we violate the principles of natural justice. One result of this can be that appeals against deregistration succeed, as they did in the case of brokers Guy Puckle, who *had* previously committed modest officially dealt with violations but who successfully appealed against the attempts in 1988 of the Securities Association to forbid them from conducting securities business.

First, the pragmatic British approach was to develop Memoranda of Understandings in which the Securities and Investments Board, as well as the Bank of England, would exchange information with banking regulators overseas whose banks had branches in Britain. Unfortunately this was not legally possible, since some countries – e.g. Liechtenstein – have laws which forbid such exchanges. Instead in Europe, letters of agreement have been signed with the Irish, French, Dutch, and Swiss banking regulators that allow more limited exchanges. In this way, the SIB accepts the right to sell securities of those firms licensed in countries whose regulatory arrangements are satisfactory to us. But subject to wider issues of commercial diplomacy and bargaining (SIB, though not a government department, is answerable to the Department of Trade and Industry, which appoints its members) this inevitably means pressure for equivalent standards and for communication of regulatory efforts transnationally, to impress other regulators with the efforts one is making to keep one's own market clean. Second, the *social* effect of regulators meeting frequently means that they can just pick up the phone with some grounded expectation of having their views listened to, unless they suspect corruption on the part of their colleagues. And third, more frequent transnational communication means that countries develop greater *expertise* in the procedures required to get information, such as mutual assistance. The fear of making a mistake – of the wheel coming off – is a great deterrent to international action in policing and non-police regulatory circles. If you do nothing it is often easier, since the consequences – if any – of doing nothing lie further in the future, by which time one may be in a different department! So as expertise develops – if staff can be retained – the internationalisation of securities regulation will increase, though the impact of such regulation on fraud is difficult to measure, since the reporting rate is unknown and even where insolvency occurs, the attribution of this to fraud is often problematical.

This discussion of the development of securities regulation has contained relatively little about *Europe*. There is a reason for this: most of the impetus for developing international co-operation has come from the US Securities and Exchange Commission (SEC), and autonomous European initiatives have been comparatively modest. They have also tended to be bilateral rather than multilateral or pan-European. One reason for this is that Europe, *qua* Europe, is engaged far more unevenly in the provision of financial services than in some other spheres such as manufacturing: London dwarfs the other European markets for securities, and the very big players are London, New York, and Tokyo. Another is that there are some differences of regulatory philosophy: the Federal Republic of Germany (FRG) requires securities traders to have large capital reserve ratios, unlike other countries such as the UK which tie capital to the amount of risk they take. It is alleged that the motive for the FRG policy is to make it a less attractive venue for foreign securities traders who do not wish to tie up their working capital unnecessarily. So as the 1989 European Directive on insider trading has demonstrated, 'harmonisation' entails war conducted by other means. Nevertheless, given our obsession with controlling illegal narcotics and terrorism, the use of banking and securities firms as conduits for 'dirty money' focuses police, media, and political attention upon financial intermediaries and creates pressure for international initiatives to regulate money flows (Anderson 1989; Walter 1989; Levi, forthcoming).

What has tended to happen is that individual countries have experienced particular pressures, and have responded to them with little regard to the problems elsewhere, though there is increasingly a search for legislative, policing and prosecutorial models to copy. Although, within Europe, it is arguable that the West Germans have the greatest expertise and organisation in dealing with economic crime, other countries have not tended to adopt their methods unchanged. To deal with financial crime, the UK has introduced draconian legislation in the Financial Services Act 1986 and the Criminal Justice Act 1987 to allow Department of Trade and Industry Inspectors and officials of the new Serious Fraud Office to require suspects and non-suspects alike to answer questions which may incriminate them (Levi 1987a). It has also reformed trial procedures and evidentiary rules in the Criminal Justice Act 1988 with the objective of making serious fraud cases easier to try. That legislation also provides for the confiscation of the assets of *convicted* fraudsters, or imprisonment in lieu of payment of assets held overseas that cannot be repatriated involuntarily, because there are no provisions for international enforcement of penal sanctions. The Dutch too have toughened up their legislation, improved the expertise of their police and prosecution departments, and have developed their interest in fraud regulation.

Yet despite the pressures towards uniformity imposed (1) by the imperatives of the globalisation of securities markets and (2) by American legal imperialism in claims to extra-territorial enforcement of its domestic legislation – of which a prime example is the Co-ordinating Committee for Export Controls (COCOM) rules that prohibit any American components in politically sensitive areas from being exported to Communist countries – this march towards heavy powers to deal with serious fraud is not universal. ('Serious fraud' is itself a term of some ambiguity, for by what criteria are we to judge seriousness? Public opinion? Size of fraud? Impact upon the economy? Impact upon the poorer sections of society?) Sometimes, constitutional factors (as in the Republic of Ireland) or national economic interests (in, say, the tax haven or banking secrecy businesses: see Levi, forthcoming) restrict the movement towards a commercial law and order society. For at the other extreme from the UK, in the Republic of Ireland, the powers of the Gardai are so restricted that they cannot interview suspects without their consent, nor without a solicitor being present, and they have no powers to seize documents.

In addition to changes in police powers, there are many developments pending regarding substantive law and the law of criminal jurisdiction, not least because there are many examples of activities considered fraudulent which the English courts have held to be outside their jurisdiction. The Law Commission (1989) has proposed to alter laws of jurisdiction so that – as in the New Zealand Crimes Act 1961 – an offence is to be regarded as having taken place in England and Wales when *any* act or event which is an essential element in the definition of the offence occurs there. This compares with the present position which is that an offence takes place within the jurisdiction of the courts only when the *last* act or even one necessary for the completion of the offence occurs here. Continental countries do not suffer from these curious principles of jurisdiction. (For a review, see Leigh 1988; Law Commission 1989.)

Developments in policing and prosecution of fraud in Europe

The fashionable trend in the control of fraud is towards inter-disciplinary team work. The West Germans began this in the 1970s, as did the Scandinavians. But local relationships are always important, and in England and Wales – though less so in Scotland where the Procurator Fiscal's interventions are, though rare, more readily legitimised (Moody and Tombs 1982) – the tradition of local constabulary independence has always inhibited the development of teamwork. Accountants could always be brought in to assist in fraud enquiries, but they cost even more money than our police and this has to be justified in budgets. But there are cultural obstacles too, arising out of some police beliefs that 'we are the professionals' and that accountants are not directed at proof of guilt, alongside the fear that if you work with accountants, your own ignorance will be revealed. Particularly where, as in the UK, assignments to Fraud Squads are seldom longer than three years on any one posting, not losing face becomes more important than learning the job properly. After all, who is to say that you have *not* done the job properly, when you can write the complaint off as 'no crime' or can blame the prosecutors or the jury for failure to take the case forward to conviction? Similar arguments apply to prosecutors, who were (and in many cases still are) generally amateurs in the prosecution of fraud. This whole process received scathing criticism in Leigh (1982), Levi (1987a), and in the Report of the Fraud Trials Committee (1986). Subsequently the Serious Fraud Office was established which again was an uneasy constitutional compromise: a body of lawyers and some few accountants was to undertake investigations and prosecutions, assisted by the police on an *ad hoc* basis (Wood 1989). The police, however, were to remain under the command of their own Chief Constables, and would be (in principle) no more expert or specialist or long-term than any other Fraud Squad officers. In practice, though, they will be directed by Serious Fraud Office lawyers, so the UK is gradually moving towards a Continental or American model of prosecutor direction of enquiries.

The French model of dealing with commercial crime remains broadly that while the police and accountants can be involved in difficult cases, the prosecutor and, even more, the *juge d'instruction* play the dominant co-ordinating role. The French – like the West Germans – have always had considerable powers to investigate, partly because their powers derive from judicial investigations. The police also investigate tax crimes on behalf of the *juges d'instruction*, and in the police *brigade financière* – whose members, unlike UK police, are generally long-term in the job – there are always attached two tax officials on secondment. Police cases are then filtered through to the prosecutor, who decides whether or not to take it to the examining magistrate. If he does *not*, the victim can always take the case to the magistrate by becoming a *partie civile*. The French have wide-ranging legislation on fraud, called *abus de biens sociaux*, about which Leigh (1984) has written cogently, which makes it an offence for directors of a company who, acting in bad faith, make a use of the assets or credit of the company which they know to be contrary to the interests of the company, either for their own personal ends or in order to favour another company or enterprise in which they are interested directly or indirectly. In France, it is relatively easy for victims to complain. Whereas neither the police nor prosecutor can examine witnesses under oath, the examining magistrate – like UK Department of Trade and Industry (DTI) inspectors and Serious Fraud Office (SFO) – can do so (though suspects are not usually so examined, because in France they cannot be sworn witnesses in their own case). The prosecutor can also grant, under letters rogatory, search and seizure powers, order electronic eavesdropping and the inspection of bank accounts and other records such as broking transactions, and commission expert witnesses. (Though in France, unlike the Federal Republic of Germany and, in SFO cases, the UK, it remains rare for accountants to be attached to an investigation directly.) Nevertheless, the expertise of examining magistrates and of judges is quite *ad hoc*, and they have little formal training or formal specialisation. Again, if one is discussing trends, it is simple logic to argue that the more cases of fraud and corporate crime that come up, the greater will be the expertise of those dealing with them, by virtue of greater experience.

The other major area of development is in respect of frauds against EC funds themselves, which have been 'guesstimated' at up to £6 billion annually. The catalogue of lax controls, waste and fraud has been amply dealt with elsewhere (Court of Auditors 1988; House of Lords 1989; Tutt 1989), and suffice it here to observe that there has been a gradual strengthening of investigators based at the Commission, whose numbers in 1989 reached double figures. But individual governments, only some of whom make net losses as a result of such frauds, still retain the primary responsibility for policing and prosecuting such frauds.

In all systems, there is some overlap between tax authorities and the more criminally oriented investigation and prosecution bodies. I say this with some irony because of course tax matters often potentially *are* criminal, but they are not treated as such, being viewed almost exclusively as administrative settlements (Cook 1989; Levi 1987a; and, for a Third World dimension, Levi and Suddle 1989). In Britain, there remains some tension between tax and police investigators, though the Serious Fraud Office is superimposed upon them and can, in theory *and* if it knows about a case, take it over from the DTI or the tax authorities or the police. Even in the Netherlands, there are parallel agencies of the police and Crown Prosecutors, on the one hand, and the *Economische Controledienst*, under the *Ministerie van Economische Zaken*, on the other. Structures may change, but personal and organisational rivalries and empire-building are features of formal organisations everywhere in the world, and when we look at abstract models in different countries, we must always be aware that harmonious interpersonal relationships, as well as formal powers, expertise, and training, are the key to successful control of economic crime.

Cartel offences

Adam Smith observed that whenever two businessmen get together, we can be sure that they are plotting some conspiracy against the public interest. Cartels – conspiracies to fix prices or to conduct other restraints on trade – are one of the oldest forms of commercial conspiracy, and action against anti-competitive practices is one area where specifically *European* policy, via the EC, has made a substantial difference to what otherwise would have been primarily *national* legislation. This can vary enormously from the FRG – which has heavy administrative penalties (Strobl *et al.* 1986) – to the UK – which has very mild civil sanctions – to Italy, which has apparently no sanctions at all. Thus, with some exceptions under Article 85(3), the Treaty of Rome prohibits conduct causing an appreciable restraint of competition that *may* affect trade between member states. There is no space here for an overview of EC law on anti-competition policy (see Tiedemann 1980; Steiner 1988; Swan 1988). During the 1980s, the Commission has become more proactive and has resorted increasingly to raiding corporate premises without advance warning to search for information regarding cartels and other unlawful agreements: the legality of such raids – of which there were eleven in 1987 – which require an administrative decision but no judicial search warrant, has been upheld by the European Court of Justice. Normally by the nature of their being able to have a substantial effect on competition, large corporations who are the principal offenders are affected by these search powers. The competition law activities of the EC are reviewed annually (European Commission 1988, 1989).

I have deliberately chosen to place cartel offences under the heading of fraud and financial crime rather than in the next section on non-fraud offences. This is because whatever the rationalisations adopted by corporate executives – e.g. that they are simply trying to stabilise the market, thereby acting in the national interest (which just happens to coincide with their own!) – cartels are in fact a kind of fraud upon competitors and upon the public who are forced to pay more for goods than they would otherwise do. The fact that large corporations are sometimes subjected to administrative or criminal measures and large fines does not tell us anything about their equal treatment compared with other offenders in Europe discussed elsewhere in this book. Those who are interested in the deliberate or unselfconscious differential treatment of crimes might reflect on the question of why without-notice raids – which are commonplace by the police in ordinary crime – excite such controversy when their targets are commercial premises, whether they are conducted by the police, revenue authorities, or other agencies (Cook 1989; Levi 1987a). The absence of prior notice seem to reflect upon the firms raided as if they were not gentlemen who could be trusted: if prior notice were adopted more generally in police investigations, perhaps this might be an excellent method of reducing the prison population.

NON-FRAUD CORPORATE CRIME CONTROL

One area that has received far less attention is the European aspect of health and safety at work and other forms of environmental offences. In view of the results of crime seriousness surveys (Miethe 1984; Levi 1987a) – which generally indicate that at least when willing or deliberate, such offences are among the most serious of *violent* crimes – this is surprising. But it is explicable partly in relation to the splitting off of responsibility from the police onto less public (and less publicity hungry) regulatory agencies, and partly because of the difficulty in attributing blame and intentionality in practice. Social harms in the late 1980s – toxic waste dumping, deaths on the railways, the sinking of the *Herald of Free Enterprise* near Zeebrugge, Piper Alpha and other North Sea explosions – reveal the difficulties entailed in defining harms as 'corporate homicide' compared with individual or group *deliberate* homicide, for irrespective of what the courts may decide, the ferry deaths were plainly not intended or wanted by Townsend Thoresen (now P&O) nor were any of the work-place deaths discussed here the product of malevolence. The social and even academic construction of the word 'violence' commonly excludes health and safety risks at work: a tradition reinforced by the *1988 British Crime Survey* (Mayhew *et al.* 1989), whose novel and interesting chapter on crime – including 'violent crime' – at work does not even mention this as a conceptual issue. (See further, Swigert and Farrell 1981; Wells 1988.) In many European countries, though not England, there are further difficulties caused by the principle that corporations cannot be criminally liable, only individuals.

There was a general drift to the political right in many European countries during the 1980s, and this was usually accompanied by a diminished stress on health and safety in favour of production. Most of the inspectorates have had their staff reduced, and despite the relative autonomy of western agencies (Kagan 1989), political signals towards diminished enthusiasm for restricting entrepreneurialism have doubtless affected regulators' approaches. One consequence – though not a logically necessary one – is disasters like the Piper Alpha oil rig, but as Carson (1981) has shown, this was inherent even in the origins of North Sea oil legislation. In other words, deregulation has started from a low existing regulatory base rate. However, there has been a tendency in the UK to make most efficient use of scarce resources by concentrating them upon high-risk, untrustworthy areas, leaving the major corporations increasingly to self-police. Given resource constraints, this may be rational, for the results of studies of corporate crime (e.g. Braithwaite 1984) tend to show that large, profitable bureaucracies do generally exhibit greater safety-consciousness, perhaps encouraged by their greater profit cushions and civil litigation-proneness. However, the combination of pressures on profit margins and reduced official surveillance is a dangerous cocktail, and could well have led to a greater amount of undetected and unprosecuted corporate crime.

CONCLUSION

Followers of Michel Foucault (1977) have sought to view penal systems as carceral archipelagos which decant 'dangerous populations' – criminals or the 'mentally ill' – involuntarily from one part of the system into others. This notion of transcarceration has not generally been applied to the control of commercial crime, partly perhaps because it has been assumed that nothing is done about it anyway. However, as argued by Levi (1987a), fraudsters have learned to operate outside national boundaries, correctly believing that multiple jurisdictions create serious problems of venue and of interest in taking action. Informants state that those who formerly ran 'boiler room' operations from Holland, in which evangelistic salespeople telephoned all over Europe to offer wonderful opportunities to get in on the groundfloor of this or that allegedly 'hot-shot' stock, were closed down by the Dutch, and moved to Belgium, where regulation was lower. But whereas transcarceration is normally viewed within the boundaries of the traditional nation-state, here, in response to national attempts to control particular forms of crime, we have both *intra*national (people move from bankruptcy fraud to credit card fraud *domestically*) and *inter*national switching – subject to barriers to entry into national and international criminal markets which include criminal skills, national languages, and contacts among police, underworld, and upperworld. It is the relationship between all these criminal and crime control networks that I think we should be exploring more in criminology than most of us have done hitherto. The AIDS and narcotics scares have prompted a welcome rebirth of ethnographic research, but this does not yet appear to be reflected in studies of serious, adult professional crime in Europe nor – *pace* Anderson's (1989) excellent examination of the *politics* of international police co-operation – studies of the methods used in controlling them.

However important formal rules are – and in this area, where the accused are sophisticated and normally can readily afford good legal advice, the rules *are* important – we must look also at policing *practice* as well as at changes in legislation. I have argued at length elsewhere (Levi 1987a, 1987b) that although they are aimed at creating an appearance of orderly honest markets so that investors will have confidence in them, it is simplistic to view fraud-related legislative changes as being *purely* symbolic. They are having real consequences and are leading to what in British terms is an unprecedented number of prosecutions of high-status individuals, even if the Serious Fraud Office has not yet made much impact upon their conviction rate. Whether such prosecutions will continue to increase is a matter for speculation, and it is hard to avoid tautological statements such as 'if the pressure to reassure investors continues, the policing and prosecutorial resources devoted to fraud will be sustained'. We do not have enough knowledge of the dynamics of regulation to specify more precisely the conditions under which this process will operate.

This relates also to one point that is equally relevant to other forms of corporate crime regulation: how do we judge the level of regulatory activity and performance? Biderman and Reiss (1967) have observed that rises in crime rates could be viewed more as an index of social progress than of social decay. Yet even in proactive areas such as corporate crime and narcotics, rises are treated unproblematically in the media as if they reflected underlying trends in misconduct. Moreover, given that much of regulatory offence policing is carried out by persuasion and warning (Hawkins 1984; Hutter 1988), and that some who wish to reduce such social harms argue that this is actually more *effective* as a method (Braithwaite 1984, 1989), how are we to interpret increased prosecutions when we see them? The traditional line taken by most liberal and radical criminologists is that prosecutions of anti-trust are *ipso facto* 'a good thing' (even if they merely legitimise capitalism), yet this may be simplistic. Furthermore, much corporate crime regulation is undertaken by compliance officers employed by firms themselves, as well as by quasi-public employees of regulatory agencies such as stock exchanges. To examine *in*formal as well as formal controls, we have to map out changes in compliance officers' and regulators' activities as well as in the activities of Fraud Squads, Serious Fraud Officer personnel, and other official groups. Business crime regulation was a notable but unfortunate omission from a recent UN study of informal crime control (UNSDRI 1988).

It may be helpful to differentiate 'the police' from other forms of civilian social control by reference to their legal monopoly over the use of force, but looking more broadly at the control of business crime, it is clear that to restrict analysis to 'the police' (or even to add non-police prosecutions but not other forms of regulatory action) is seriously misleading. The regulation of health and safety at work remains a nation-based Cinderella service within the EC, though in the field of environmental crime, the 'greening' of all political parties and the effects of toxic waste can be expected to lead to greater attempts than hitherto at cross-border governmental monitoring and to more regulations. It remains moot, however, whether possible future requirements that all countries dispose of their own toxic waste will lead to that happening or to more *il*legal internal and cross-border dumping, perhaps by organised crime groups as in the USA (Block and Scarpitti 1985). The approach of 1992, as well as market-place pressures, has made regulatory developments regarding banking and securities fraud proceed quickly towards communal vetting of fitness and propriety, including the information flow upon which such vetting depends. Primary prevention, as well as more active central review by EC fraud investigators, will proceed in action against fraud in the EC agricultural subsidies sector. But in other spheres of business crime, attempts at control are still primarily local or national in character. There is enough difficulty getting different UK forces to co-operate with each other, without expecting the transition to trans-European fraud policing to be effected without a great deal of pain. So although to the paranoid, the International, or at least European, Police State approaches, there is as yet little evidence of its arrival in the sphere of business crime control. (Perhaps, as with the Mafia, the less hard evidence one can find, the clearer the proof of its sinister penetration.) Some may not be surprised that the policing of misconduct by corporations is loosely regulated, and that the greatest level of protection against fraud lies in the realm of small investor protection, where the political consequences of fraud are most serious. But it should not be forgotten that much of the financial fraud which occurs is at the expense of big business élites, not for their benefit, so this low level of international harmonisation of fraud control is not unambiguously in the interests of 'the powerful'.

© 1991 Michael Levi

GLOSSARY

abus de biens sociaux	abuse of social welfare
asportation crimes	crimes which involve the taking away of property, e.g. autotheft, burglary, robbery
brigade financière	financial police
comity	rules based on civilised friendship and mutual respect
commissions rogatoires	information requested from suspects and/or witnesses overseas, to be supplied by overseas police forces
'hot shot stock'	a share that is claimed by vendors to be 'guaranteed' to rise
juges d'instruction	examining magistrates
partie civile	party to a civil action
Ministerie van Economische Zaken	Ministry of Economic Affairs

Notes

CHAPTER FOUR CRIME IN EASTERN EUROPE

1 This chapter was written 1988 and edited in mid-1989, before the major changes in eastern Europe, and particularly in the GDR, took place.

CHAPTER SIX DRUGS, CRIME AND LAW ENFORCEMENT: SOME ISSUES FOR EUROPE

1 This is a revised version of a paper originally presented by the second author to the ISTD conference on 'Crime in Europe', University of York, 11–14 September 1988.
2 The paper deals only with *illicit* drug use. It is acknowledged throughout Europe – east and west – that problems relating to alcohol, tobacco and tranquilliser use are more widespread and probably far more serious; however, these cannot be dealt with here.
3 Personal communication, National Drugs Intelligence Unit, Scotland Yard, September 1989.
4 In terms of research and informed policy-making, one obvious problem at present is the language barrier. Any commitment to improved scientific dialogue on drug problems in Europe must include the dissemination of translations of national research summaries as well as the bringing together of researchers from different countries.
5 The interviews were carried out as part of a continuing study of the interaction between developments in drug-related law enforcement and legislation and changes in the drug distribution system and markets. Discussion of some aspects of the study can be found in Dorn and South 1990a and 1990b, and in Dorn *et al.* 1990. The study will be reported as Dorn, Murji and South (1991) *Policing the Drug Distribution Business*, London: Routledge.
6 Of course, treaties with other countries outside Europe have also been signed or are under negotiation.

CHAPTER TEN A TOUCH OF DISCIPLINE: ACCOUNTABILITY AND DISCIPLINE IN PRISON SYSTEMS IN WESTERN EUROPE

1 The study on which this chapter is based was funded by the UK ESRC, grant number 00232186. At the time of the study (1986–8) I was working at the University of Bath, UK. I would also like to acknowledge the help and support during the research of the following organisations: in England and Wales, the Home Office Prison Department and HORPU; in France, the Ministère de la Justice Direction de l'Administration Penitentiaire and CESDIP; in the Netherlands, the Ministerie van Justitie Directie Gevangeniswezen and the WODC; in the Federal Republic of Germany, the Justizministerium Baden-Württemberg, Justizministerium Hessen, and the Max-Planck-Institute, Freiburg im Breisgau. Responsibility for inaccuracies is mine.

2 The fieldwork on which this chapter draws comprised visits to two establishments in England, four in France, two (plus a 'satellite' of one of them) in the FRG, and three (two of which were divided into several separate sections) in the Netherlands. In each establishment a small number of staff and inmates were interviewed, though the numbers do not amount to a statistically useful sample and qualitative rather than quantitative data were collected. In all countries, visits were made to ministries of justice (in the FRG to two Länder ministries but not to the Federal ministry) and officials interviewed. Finally, academics and researchers in each country were interviewed, literature searches conducted, and unpublished data and files consulted in the ministries and prisons.

3 The rules referred to here are: in England, Prison Rule 47; in France, Code de Procedure Penale, Troisième Partie, Art D241, D242, D243, D244, D245; in the Netherlands, Beginselenwet Gevangeniswezen 32 and 45, Gevangenismaatregel (GM) 28, 49(1–2) and 100(1–5), Huishoudelijk Reglement (HR) iii 1; in the FRG, Strafvollzugsgesetz ss 37, 41, 81, 82.

4 Boards of Visitors are charged with a number of duties, including the hearing of serious disciplinary cases, the authorisation of segregation and a general oversight of the prison to which they are appointed. Their membership covers a wide spread of occupations though most members are middle class. For further discussion see Maguire and Vagg (1984).

5 The *juge de l'application des peines* has no duty to hear complaints as such. A *juge de l'application des peines* is appointed for each prison. The powers of the *juge* include decisions on remission, some parole decisions, home leave, suspension and part-suspension of sentence, and advice on various topics to the prison governor. Details may be found in the CPP, Article 720 *et seq*, and Articles D115 – 117-1, D170, D176, D180, D249, D250-1, D573 *et seq*.

6 Thus, claims that the governor followed the regulations are not in themselves a defence. The administrative regulations can themselves be determined as incompatible with the law.

Bibliography

Adler, F. (1975) *Sisters in Crime*, New York: McGraw-Hill.

—— (ed.) (1984) *The Incidence of Female Criminality in the Contemporary World*, New York: New York University Press.

Adler, F. and Simon, R. (eds) (1979) *The Criminology of Deviant Women*, Boston, Mass: Houghton Mifflin.

Advisory Council on the Misuse of Drugs (ACMD) (1984) *Prevention*, London: HMSO.

Albrecht, H.-J. (1987a) 'Foreign minorities and the criminal justice system in the Federal Republic of Germany', *Howard Journal of Criminal Justice* 26: 272–86.

—— (1987b) 'Particular difficulties in enforcing the law arising out of basic conflicts between the different agencies with regard to the best-suited reaction upon highly sensitive kinds of crime', in Council of Europe (ed.) *Interactions within the Criminal Justice System*, Strasbourg: Council of Europe.

—— (1988a) 'Ausländerkriminalität', in H. Jung (ed.) *Fälle zum Wahlfach Kriminologie, Jugendstrafrecht, Strafvollzug*, Munich: Beck.

—— (1988b) 'Strafzumessung im Vergleich Deutschland/Österreich', unpublished manuscript, Freiburg.

—— (1989a) 'Comparative research on crime and delinquency – The role and relevance of national penal codes and criminal justice systems', in M.W. Klein (ed.) *Cross-National Research in Self-Reported Crime and Delinquency*, Dordrecht/Boston/London: Kluwer.

—— (1989b) 'Ethnic minorities, crime and public policy', in R. Hood (ed.) *Crime and Criminal Policy in Europe*, Oxford: Centre for Criminological Research.

Albrecht, P.A. and Pfeiffer, Ch. (1979) *Die Kriminalisierung junger Ausländer*, Munich: Juventa.

Alderson, J. (1989) *Off the Treadmill*, BBC series on criminal justice in Europe, August.

Allen, H. (1987) *Justice Unbalanced*, Milton Keynes: Open University Press.

Andel, H. van (1989) 'Crime prevention that works: the case of public transport in the Netherlands', *British Journal of Criminology* 29, 1: 47–56.

Anderson, M. (1989) *Policing the World: Interpol and the Politics of*

International Police Co-operation, Oxford: Clarendon Press.
Andersson, J. (1984) 'Policing in multi-ethnic areas in Stockholm', in J. Brown (ed.) *Policing and Social Policy*, London: Police Review Publishing.
Antilla I. (1984) 'Female criminality in Finland – what do the statistics show?' in F. Adler (ed.) *The Incidence of Female Criminality in the Contemporary World*, New York: New York University Press.
Archer, D. and Gartner, R. (1984) *Violence and Crime in Cross-National Perspective*, New Haven, Conn: Yale University Press.
Arnold, H. (1983) 'Vorläufige Ergebnisse einer viktimologischen Untersuchung in Baden-Württemberg', unpublished manuscript, Freiburg.
Arnold, H. and Korinek, L. (1985) 'Kriminalitätsbelastung in der Bundesrepublik Deutschland und in Ungarn: Ergebnisse einer international vergleichenden Opferbefragung', in A. Bohm, H. Echert, W. Feuerhelm, F. Hamburger and G. Sander (eds) *Kriminologie in den sozialistischen Ländern*, Bochum.
Aromaa, K., Toïnudd, P., and Wartioraana, K. (1970) *Department Store Shoplifters*, Helsinki: Patrik Institute of Criminology
Aronowitz, A.A. (1989) *Assimilation, Acculturation and Juvenile Delinquency Among Second Generation Turkish Youth in Berlin, West Germany*, Albany, NY: State University of New York.
Ashworth, A. (1988) 'Criminal justice and the criminal process', in Paul Rock (ed.) *A History of British Criminology*, Oxford: Oxford University Press.
Auld, J., Dorn, N. and South, N. (1986) 'Irregular work, irregular pleasures: heroin in the 1980s', in R. Matthews and J. Young (eds) *Confronting Crime*, London: Sage.
Austin, R.L. (1981) 'Liberation and female criminality in England and Wales', *British Journal of Criminology* 21, 4: 371–4.
Barnes, M. (1981) 'The Secret Cold War: the C.I.A. and American foreign policy in Europe 1946–1956 Part I', *Historical Journal* 24: 399–415.
—— (1982) 'The Secret Cold War: the C.I.A. and American foreign policy in Europe 1946–1956 Part II', *Historical Journal* 25: 649–70.
Bärtling, Th., Jung, H., and Bärtling, K. (1982) 'Schwangerschaftskonflikt und Schwangerschaftsabbruch in ausländischen Arbeitnehmerfamilien', in H. Poettgen (ed.) *Die ungewollte Schwangerschaft*, Cologne: Deutscher Arzte Verlag.
Bennett, T. (1988) 'An assessment of the design, implementation and effectiveness of neighbourhood watch in London', *Howard Journal of Criminal Justice* 27, 4: 241–55.
Bericht der Bundesregierung über die innere Sicherheit in Osterreich (1987) Vienna: National Government of Austria.
Bibal, D., Fize, M., and Menis, D. (1985) *Les Femmes en Prison*, Paris: Ministry of Justice.
Biderman, A. and Reiss, A. (1967) 'On exploring the dark figure of crime', *Annals of the American Academy of Political and Social Science*, 374: 1–15.
Bielefeld, U. *et al.* (1982) *Junge Ausländer im Konflikt. Lebenssituationen und Überlebensformen*, Munich: Juventa.

Blaauw, J.A. (1974) De bestrijding van de georganiseerde misdaad in Nederland, *Algemeen Politieblad* 123, 10: 227–36.

Blankenburg, E. (1973) 'Die Selektivität strafrechtlicher Sanktionen', in J. Friedrichs (ed.) *Teilnehmende Beobachtung abweichenden Verhaltens*, Stuttgart: Enke.

Block. A. and Scarpitti, F. (1985) *Poisoning for Profit*, New York: William Morrow.

Blum, R. (1967) 'Mind-altering drugs and dangerous behaviour: narcotics', in President's Commission on Law Enforcement and Administration of Justice, *Task Force Report: Narcotics and Drug Abuse*, Washington, DC: US Government Printing Office.

Boge, H. (1985) 'Neue Entwicklungen des Terrorismus', *Kriminalistik*, 12: 587–92.

Bottoms, A.E. (1983) 'Some neglected features of contemporary penal systems', in D. Garland and D. Young (eds) *The Power to Punish*, London: Heinemann.

Bottoms A.E., Mawby, R., and Walker, M. (1987) 'A localised crime survey in contrasting areas of a city', *British Journal of Criminology* 27, 2: 125–54.

Bottoms, A.E. and Wiles, P. (1988) 'Urban areas, social change and crime', paper presented to the American Society of Criminology Annual Meeting, Chicago, November.

Box, S. and Hale, C. (1983) 'Liberation and female criminality in England and Wales', *British Journal of Criminology* 23, 1: 35–49.

Braithwaite, J. (1984) *Corporate Crime in the Pharmaceutical Industry*, London: Routledge.

—— (1989) *Crime, Shame and Reintegration*, Oxford: Oxford University Press.

Brantingham, P.L. and Brantingham, P.J. (1981) 'Notes on the geometry of crime', in P.J. Brantingham and P.L. Brantingham (eds) *Environmental Criminology*, Beverly Hills, Calif.: Sage.

Brown, C. (1984) *Black and White Britains: The Third PSI Survey*, Aldershot: Gower.

Bruggeman, W. and Luypaers, P. (1986) 'Autodiefstal, holdup en terrorisme in België (deel II)', *Panopticon* 7, 6: 570–81.

Brugger (1981) 'Interpol am Scheideweg?', *Die Deutsche Polizei* 9: 7–8.

Bruinsma, G.J.N., Dessaur, C.I., and Van Hezewijk, R.W.I.V. (1984) 'Female criminality in the Netherlands', in F. Adler (ed.) *The Incidence of Female Criminality in the Contemporary World*, New York: New York University Press.

Buchholz, E. (1987) 'Reasons for the low rate of delinquency in the German Demokratic Republic', in B. Holyst (ed.) *Eurocriminology*, vol. I, Warsaw: Polish Scientific Publishers.

Buckle, A. and Farrington, D. (1984) 'An observational study of shoplifting', *British Journal of Criminology* 24, 1: 63–73.

Bundeskriminalamt (ed.) (1985) *Ausgewahlte Zahlen für die Rechts pflege Reihel*, Wiesbaden: Bundeskriminalamt.

—— (1987) *Polizeiliche Kriminalstatistik 1986* (English summary), Wiesbaden: Bundeskriminalamt.

Bundesministerium der Justiz (ed.) (1988) *Schadenswiedergutmachung im*

Kriminalrecht, Bonn: Untersuchung des Fachausschusses I 'Strafrecht und Strafvollzug' des Bundesverbandes der Straffälligenhilfe e.V. Bonn.

Burke, H., Carney, C., and Cooke, G. (eds) (1981) *Youth and Justice*, Dublin: Turoe Press.

Cain, M. (ed.) (1989) *Growing Up Good*, London: Sage.

Cario, R. (1985) 'La Criminalité des femmes: approche differentielle', Université de Pau et des Pays de L'Adur, thèse pour Dr d'Etat, 22 Fevrier.

—— (1987) 'Contribution à la commissance et à l'explication de la criminalité des femmes', *Revue Internat de Criminologie et de Police Technique*, 3: 306–30.

Carlen, P. (1983) *Women's Imprisonment*, London: Routledge & Kegan Paul.

Carlen, P. (1985) *Criminal Women*, Cambridge: Polity.

Carlen, P. and Worrall, A. (eds) (1987) *Gender, Crime and Justice*, Milton Keynes: Open University Press.

Carr-Hill, R.A. (1987) 'O bring me your poor: immigrants in the French system of criminal justice', *Howard Journal of Criminal Justice* 26: 287–302.

Carson, W. (1981) *The Other Price of Britain's Oil*, Oxford: Martin Robertson.

Central Bureau of Statistics of Norway (1988) Oslo: Criminal Statistics 1986.

Christiansen, K.O. (1974) 'Seriousnes of criminality and concordance among Danish twins', in R. Hood (ed.) *Crime, Criminology and Public Policy*, London: Heinemann.

Christiansen, K.O. (1977) 'A preliminary study of criminality among twins', in S. Mednick and K.O. Christiansen (eds) *Biosocial Bases of Criminal Behaviour*, New York: Gardener.

Cohen, S. (1985) *Visions of Social Control*, Cambridge: Polity.

Colder, J.C. (1988) *Het winkelcentraproject: preventie van kleine criminaliteit*, The Hague: Government Printing Office.

Commission of the European Communities (1988) *Social Europe*, Luxembourg.

Cook, D. (1989) *Rich Law, Poor Law*, Milton Keynes: Open University Press.

Cooper, H.H.A. (1979) 'Woman as terrorist', in F. Adler and R. Simon (eds) *The Criminology of Deviant Women*, Boston, Mass: Houghton Mifflin.

Council of Europe (1981) *Economic Crime*, Strasbourg: Council of Europe.

—— (1985) *Recommendation on the Position of the Victim in the Framework of Criminal Law and Procedure*, R. (85) 11, Strasbourg: Council of Europe.

—— (1986) Parliamentary Assembly, Legal Affairs Committee, *Draft Report on International Crime* (submitted by Mr Stoffelen, *Rapporteur*), AS/Jur. (38) 14 Part II.

—— (1987) *Recommendation on the Organisation of Crime Prevention*, R. (87) 19, Strasbourg: Council of Europe.

—— (1988a) *Prison Information Bulletin* 11, June: 18–20.

—— (1988b) *Prison Information Bulletin* 12, December.

Court of Auditors (1988) 'Annual report concerning the financial year 1987', *Official Journal of the European Communities*, 31, C316.

Craen, A. (1984) 'Policing and social policy in multi-ethnic areas of Ghent', in J. Brown (ed.) *Policing and Social Policy*, London: Police Review Publishing.

Cremer-Schäfer, H. (1988) 'Modernisierung der Kontrolle in der Nachkriegszeit', *Kriminologische Bibliographie*, 15: 68–84.

Crow, I. (1987) 'Black people and criminal justice in the UK', *Howard Journal of Criminal Justice* 26: 303–14.

Currie, E. (1988) 'Two visions of community crime prevention', in T. Hope and M. Shaw (eds) *Communities and Crime Reduction*, London: HMSO.

Die Waage – Köln (1987) *Jahresbericht*, Annual Report of the Waage Projekt, Köln.

Dit Commentaar op de Benelux is ontleend aan een niet-gepubliceerd manuscript van een vergelijkende studie over het Belgische en Nederlandse politiewezen.

Dobash, R.P., Dobash, R.E., and Gutteridge, S. (1986) *The Imprisonment of Women*, Oxford: Blackwell.

Dorn, N., Murji, K., and South, N. (1990) 'Mirroring the market?: current debates on police effectiveness and reorganisation to defeat drug trafficking', in R. Reiner and M. Cross (eds) *Beyond Law and Order*, London: Macmillan.

—— (1991) *Policing the Drug Distribution Business*, London: Routledge.

Dorn, N. and South, N. (1990a) 'Profits and penalities: new trends in legislation and law enforcement concerning illegal drugs', in D. Whynes and P. Bean (eds) *Policing and Prescribing: The British System of Drug Control*, London: Macmillan.

—— (1990b) 'Drug markets and law enforcement', *British Journal of Criminology*, in press.

Downes, D. (1988) *Contrasts in Tolerance*, Oxford: Clarendon Press.

—— (ed.) (1989) *Crime and the City*, Basingstoke: Macmillan.

Druglink (1989a) Various articles on crack, *Druglink*, September/October: whole issue.

—— (1989b) 'Regional anti-drug campaigns', Druglink, July/August: 10–11.

Dubois, J.P. (1978) 'Le Marché Commun contre les libertés' *Journal des Juristes Democrates* 1: 11–14.

Duft, H., Heilborn, H., Müller, R., Pruss, U., Schlegel, J., Teichler, G., and Weber, H. (eds) (1981) *Strafrecht der Deutschen Demokratischen Republik. Kommentar zum Strafgesetzbuch*, Staatsverlag der Deutschen Demokratischen Republik, Berlin.

Dutch Social and Cultural Planning Report (1986), Rijksivijk: Dutch Social and Cultural Office.

Dyson, K. (1980) *The State Tradition in Western Europe*, Oxford: Martin Robertson.

Eaton, M. (1986) *Justice for Women?* Milton Keynes: Open University Press.

Einsele, H. (1981) 'Female criminality in the Federal Republic of Germany', Strasbourg: Council of Europe.

Elmhorn, K. (1969) *Faktisk Brottslighet Bland Skolbarn*, Stockholm: Statens Offentliga Utreduingar.

Enhus, E. and Hendrieckx, C. (1988) *La Relation Police Public*, Brussels: Vrije Universiteit Brussels.

European Commission (1988) *Seventeenth Report on Competition Policy*, Luxembourg: Commission of the European Communities.

—— (1989) *Eighteenth Report on Competition Policy*, Luxembourg: Commission of the European Communities.

European Parliament Working Documents (1986–7) A-Series, Document A 2-114/86/Corr. *Report Drawn up on Behalf of the Committee of Enquiry into the Drugs Problem in the Member States of the Community on the Results of the Enquiry*, Strasbourg.

Fattah, E. (ed.) (1986) *From Crime Policy to Victim Policy*, London: Macmillan.

Faugeron, C. (1989) 'Crime prevention policy: current state and prospects; a commentary', in *Proceedings II European Colloquium on Crime and Public Policy in Europe*, Freiburg: Max-Planck-Institute.

Faugeron, C. and Houchon, G. (1987) 'Towards a sociology of penal policy', *International Journal of the Sociology of Law* 15: 393–422.

Faugeron, C. and Rivero, N. (1982) *Femmes libérées sous condition*, Paris: Ministère de la Justice.

Feest, J. (1985) 'Fraunenkriminalität' in G. Kaiser *et al.* (eds) *Kleines Kriminologisches Wörterbuch*, Heidelberg: Müller.

—— (1988) ' "Prisoners" rights in Germany: legislation, implementation and evaluation', paper presented at a conference on 'Aspects of European Criminal and Penal Policy', Bristol, 30 January.

Fenyó, A. (1975) 'The Hungarian penal system after the liberation', in *Development of the Political and Legal System of the Hungarian People's Republic in the Past 30 Years*, Hungarian Lawyers' Association.

Ferand, H. and Schlanitz (1975) 'La coopération policière internationale', *Revue Internationale de Droit Pénal*, Numéro Spécial: 475–97.

Ferrari-Bravo, G. and Arcidiacono, C. (1989) 'Compounded misunderstanding: relations between staff and girls in an Italian prison', in M. Cain (ed.) *Growing Up Good*, London: Sage.

Field, F. (1989) *Losing Out*, Oxford: Blackwell.

Field, S. and Hope, T. (1989) 'Economics, the consumer and underprovision in crime prevention', extended version of an article in *Home Office Research and Planning Unit Research Bulletin* 26: 40–4.

Fijnaut, C.J.C. (1982) 'The limits of direct police cooperation in Western Europe', *Police Studies* 5, 3: 52–7.

—— (1983) *De zaak François: beschouwingen naar aanleiding van het vonnis*, Antwerpen: Kluwer Rechtswetenschappen, pp. 5–43.

—— (1985) 'Georganiseerde misdaad: een onderzoeksgerichte terreinverkenning', *Justitiële Verkenningen* 8: 5–42.

—— (1986) 'De politiële bestrijding van politiek terrorisme in Westelijk Europa', *Nieuw Europa* 12, 2: 48–53.

—— (1987) 'The internationalization of criminal investigation in Western Europe', in C.J.C. Fijnaut and R. Hermans (eds) *Police Co-operation in Europe*, Lochem: J.B. van den Brink.

Fijnaut, C.J.C. and Hermans, R. (eds) (1987) *Police Co-operation in Europe*, Lochem: J.B. van den Brink.

Fijnaut, C.J.C., Nuijten-Edelbroek, E.G.M., and Spickenheuer, J.L.P. (1985) *Politiële misdaadbestrijding: de ontwikkeling van het Amerikaanse, Engelse en Nederlandse onderzoek aangaande politiële misdaadbestrijding sedert de jaren '60*, 's-Gravenhage: Staatsuitgeverij.

Fijnaut, C.J.C. and Visser, B. (eds) (1985) *Managing Larger Police Organizations*, Amsterdam: Municipal Police Force.

Fitzgerald, E. (1985) 'Prison discipline and the courts', in M. Maguire, J. Vagg, and R. Morgan (eds) *Accountability and Prisons: Opening up a Closed World*, London: Tavistock.

Folgesvold and Dullum (1988) Personal communication.

Fontanesi, M. (1980) *Women's Criminality in Italy*, Strasbourg: Council of Europe.

Foucault, M. (1977) *Discipline and Punish*, London: Allen Lane.

Fowler, F., MacCalla, M.E., and Mangione, T.W. (1979) *Reducing Residential Crime and Fear: The Hartford Neighborhood Crime Prevention Program*, Washington, DC: US Government Printing Office.

Frankowski, S.J. (1987) 'Poland', in G.F. Cole, S.J. Frankowski, and M.G. Gertz (eds) *Major Criminal Justice Systems*, 2nd edn, Newbury Park/ Beverly Hills/London/New Delhi: Sage.

Fraud Trials Committee (1986) *Report*, London: HMSO.

Frost and Sullivan Ltd (1988) *Residential Security Markets in Western Europe, 1988*, London: Frost and Sullivan.

Garrison, O.V. (n.d.) *The Secret World of Interpol*, New York: Ralston Pilot Inc., s.d.

Gelsthorpe, L. and Morris, A. (1988) 'Feminism and criminology in Britain', *British Journal of Criminology* 28, 2: 93–110.

Genders, E. and Player, E. (1986) 'Women's imprisonment: the effects of youth custody', *British Journal of Criminology* 26, 4: 357–71.

Graham, J. (1988) 'Crime prevention in the Federal Republic of Germany', *Home Office Research and Planning Unit Research Bulletin* 24: 37–41.

—— (1989) 'Crime prevention: a pan European perspective', paper given to ISTD Conference on 27 November.

—— (1990a) *Manual of Crime Prevention*, Helsinki: HEUNI.

—— (1990b) 'Reducing the West German prison population', *British Journal of Criminology* 30, 2: 150–70.

Greger, R. (1987) 'Strafzumessung bei Vergewaltigung', *Monatsschrift für Kriminologie und Strafrechtsreform* 70: 261–77.

Gruner, R. (1974) 'Vorschläge zur Realisierung des Europol – Gedankens', in Bund Deutscher Kriminalbeamter, *Europäische Gemeinschaft – auch für die Kriminalpolizei? Berichtsheft zur zweiten Fachtagung 'Kripo International 74'*, Berlin: 16–20.

Gulbinowicz, D. (1978) 'The International Criminal Police Organization', unpublished manuscript, City University of New York.

Hagan, J. (1977) *The Disreputable Pleasures*, Toronto: McGraw-Hill.

Hagemann-White, C. (1981) *Hilfen für mißhandelte Frauen*, Stuttgart: Enke.

Hailbronner, E. (1984) *Ausländerrecht*, Munich: C.F. Müller.

Hanak, G. (1987) 'Ethnographie der Konfliktbearbeitung', *Kriminalsoziologische Bibliographie* 14: 9–34.

Hanak, G., Pilgram, A., and Stangel, W. (1984) 'Die Strafverfolgung an Ausländern – Eine Sekundärauswertung zweier soziologischer Studien zur Rechtsanwendung', *Kriminalsoziologische Bibliographie* 11: 41–53.

Hanak, G., Stehr, J., and Steinert, H. (1989) *Ärgernisse und Lebenskatastrophen: Über den alltäglichen Umgang mit Kriminalität*, Bielefeld: AJZ.

Hansard (1989) 'Drug abuse', *Hansard*, Westminster, 9 June: 522–3.

Hartnoll, R. (1986) 'Current situation relating to drug abuse assessment in European countries', *Bulletin on Narcotics* 38, 1/2: 65–80.

—— (1989) 'The international context', in S. MacGregor (ed.) *Drugs and British Society*, London: Routledge.

Hawkins, K. (1984) Environment and Enforcement, Oxford: Clarendon Press.

Heckmann, F. (1983) 'Towards a typology of minorities', in C. Fried (ed.) *Minorities: Community and Identity*, Berlin/Heidelberg/New York/Tokyo: Springer.

Heidensohn, F.M. (1968) 'The deviance of women: a critique and an enquiry', *British Journal of Sociology* 19(2): 160–75.

—— (1985) *Women and Crime*, London: Macmillan.

—— (1987) 'Women and crime: questions for Criminology', in P. Carlen and A. Worrall (eds) *Gender, Crime and Justice*, Milton Keynes: Open University Press.

Heine, G. and Meinberg, V. (1989) 'Environmental criminal law in Europe', paper given to II European Colloquium on Crime and Criminal Policy in Europe, to be published by the Max-Planck-Institute, Freiburg.

Herold, H. (1974) 'Zielvorstellungen für die Verbrechensbekämpfung in der EG', in Bund Deutscher Kriminalbeamter *Europäische Gemeinschaft – auch für die Kriminalpolizei? Berichtsheft zur zweiten Fachtagung 'Kripo International 74'*, Berlin: 28–33.

—— (1980) 'Informationssysteme in der internationalen Verbrechensbekämpfung: Entwicklungsstand und Perspektiven', in Bundesvorstand des Bund Deutscher Kriminalbeamter *Grenzüberschreitende Verbrechensbekämpfung in Spiegelbild zwischenstaatlicher Verträge und gesetzlicher Regelungen*, Berlin.

Herrmann, J. (1987) 'The Federal Republic of Germany', in G.F. Cole, S.J. Frankowski, and M.G. Gertz (eds) *Major Criminal Justice Systems*, 2nd edn, Newbury Park/Beverly Hills/London/New Delhi: Sage.

HEUNI (1985) *Criminal Justice Systems in Europe: Report of the Ad Hoc Expert Group on a Cross-National Study on Trends in Crime and Information Sources on Criminal Justice and Crime Prevention in Europe*, Helsinki: HEUNI.

Høigård, C. and Snare, A. (1983) *Kvimers Skyld*, Oslo: Bakgater.

Holyst, B. (1979) *Comparative Criminology*, Toronto: Lexington Books.

Home Office (1981) *Racial Attacks*, London: HMSO.

—— (1985a) *Tackling Drug Misuse: A Summary of the Government's Strategy*, 1st edn, London: HMSO.

—— (1985b) *Report of the Departmental Committee on the Prison Disciplinary System*, 2 vols, 'Prior Report', London: HMSO.

—— (1986) *Criminal Statistics*, London: Home Office.

—— (1987) *Special European Edition: Crime Prevention in Europe*, Research Bulletin, London: Home Office.

—— (1988a) *The Costs of Crime*, London: Home Office.

—— (1988b) *Report of the Working Group on the Costs of Crime*, Standing Conference on Crime Prevention, London: Home Office.

Hood, R. (1989) *Crime and Criminal Policy in Europe*, Oxford: Centre for Criminological Research, University of Oxford.

Hope, T. and Shaw, M. (1988a) 'Community approaches to reducing crime', in T. Hope and M. Shaw (eds) *Communities and Crime Reduction*, London: HMSO.

—— (eds) (1988b) *Communities and Crime Reduction*, London: HMSO.

Hough, M. and Mayhew, P. (1983) *The British Crime Survey: First Report*, London: HMSO.

House of Lords (1989) *Fraud Against the Community*, 5th Report of the Select Committee on the European Community, HL Paper 27-1, London: HMSO.

Huins, J.M.M. (1980) 'Need for effective international police co-operation in the fight against increasing international crime: an examination of the effectiveness of Interpol in fulfilling the needs of the United Kingdom at the approach of the 1980s', unpublished manuscript, Bramshill: Police Staff College.

Humphrey, D. (1972) *Police Power and Black People*, London.

Hutter, B. (1988) *The Reasonable Arm of the Law*, Oxford: Clarendon Press.

Ignatieff, M. (1978) *A Just Measure of Pain*, New York: Pantheon.

Interpol (1986) 'The drug problem; the situation in Europe (1983–4)', *International Criminal Police Review* 395: 46–54.

—— (1987) 'International drug traffic', *International Criminal Police Review* 409: 17–20.

Jager, J. (1989) *Gewalt in unseren Städten als Beispiel für Aufgaben der Kommunalen Kriminalpolitik*, Internationales Kolloquium 26–30 September 1988, Münster: Polizei-Führungakademie.

Jahresbericht die Waage (1987) Annual Report of the Waage-Projekt, Cologne.

Jeffery, C.R. (1977) *Crime Prevention through Environmental Design*, Beverly Hills, Calif: Sage.

Jehle, J. (1985) *Untersuchungshaft zwischen Unschuldsvermutung und Wiedereingliederung*, Munich: Minerva.

Jenkins, J. (1989) 'Foreign exchange', *New Statesman and Society*, 28 July: 12–13.

Jensen, A. (1984) 'Norwegian women in court', in F. Adler (ed.) *The Incidence of Female Criminality in the Contemporary World*, New York: New York University Press.

Jeschke, J. (1980) 'Gegenwart und Zukunft der IKPO-Interpol', in Bundesvorstand des Bundes Deutscher Kriminalbeamter *Grenzüberschreitende Verbrechensbekämpfung im Spiegelbild zwischenstaatlicher Verträge und gesetzlicher Regelungen*, Berlin: 14–28.

Johnson, B., Goldstein, P., Preble, E., Scmeidler, J., Lipton, D., Spunt, B., and Miller, T. (1985) *Taking Care of Business: The Economics of Crime by Heroin Users*, Lexington, Mass: Lexington Books.

Johnson, E.H. (1987) *Handbook on Crime and Delinquency Prevention*, New York: Greenwood Press.

Jones, T., Maclean, B. and Young, J. (1986) *The Islington Crime Survey: Crime, Victimization and Policing in Inner-City London*, Aldershot: Gower.

Joutsen, M. (1987) *The Role of the Victim of Crime in European Criminal Justice Systems*, Helsinki Institute for Crime Prevention and Control series no. 11, Helsinki: HEUNI.

Jung, H. (ed.) (1989) *Alternativen zur Strafjustiz und die Garantie individueller Rechte der Betroffenen: Participatory Models and Individual Rights*, Bonn: Forum Verlag.

Junger, M. (1989) 'Ethnic minorities, crime and public policy', in R. Hood (ed.) *Crime and Criminal Policy in Europe*, Oxford: Centre for Criminological Research, University of Oxford.

Junger, M. and von Hecke, T. (1988) *Schadevergoeding binnen het Strafrecht. Daders en slachtoffers van Misdrijven*, The Hague: Ministry of Justice.

Junger-Tas, J. (1981) *Politiecontacten van minderjarigen en justitielle afdoening*, The Hague: Ministry of Justice.

—— (1984a) 'Minority juveniles and the Dutch police', in J. Brown (ed.) *Policing and Social Policy*, London: Police Review Publishing.

—— (1984b) *Recent Trends in Juvenile Delinquency*, The Hague: Ministry of Justice.

—— (1985) *Young Immigrants in the Netherlands and their Contacts with the Police*, The Hague: Ministry of Justice.

Junger-Tas, J. and Block, R. (1988) *Juvenile Delinquency in the Netherlands*, Amstelveen, the Netherlands: Kugler.

Just, W.-D. and Groth, A. (1985) *Wanderarbeiter in der EG*, Mainz: Grünewald.

Kagan, R. (1989) 'Understanding regulatory enforcement', *Law and Policy* 11, 2: 89–120.

Kaiser, G. (1988) *Kriminologie, Ein Lehrbuch: 2, völlig neubearbeitete und erweiterte Auflage*, Heidelberg: C.F. Müller Juristicher Verlag.

Kaiser, G., Kerner, H-J., and Schöch, H. (1983) *Strafvollzug*, Heidelberg: C.F. Müller.

Kaiser, G. and Metzger-Pregizer, G. (eds) (1976) *Betriebsjustiz*, Berlin: Duncker & Humblodt.

Karger, Th. and Sutterer, P. (1988) 'Cohort study on the development of police recorded criminality and criminal sanctioning', in G. Kaiser and I. Geissler (eds) *Crime and Criminal Justice*, Freiburg: Max-Planck-Institute.

Kersten, J. (1989) 'The institutional control of girls and boys', in M. Cain (ed.) *Growing Up Good*, London: Sage.

Killias, M. (1988) 'Diskriminierendes Anzeigeverhalten von Opfern gegenüber Ausländern?', *Monatsschrift für Kriminologie und Strafrechtsreform* 71: 156–65.

—— (1989) *Les Suisses face au crime*, Grusch, Switzerland: Ruegger.

King, R.D. and McDermott, K. (1989) 'British prison 1970–1987: the ever-deepening crisis', *British Journal of Criminology* 29, 2: 107–28.

Klink, M. (1987) 'Die Zusammenarbeit europäischer Polizeien in Sicherheitsfragen', *Die Polizei* 78, 7: 183–9.

Koch, I. (1983) 'Krinder î faengsel', in C. Høigård and A. Snare (eds) *Kvinners Skyld*, Oslo: Bakgater.

Körner, H. and Mehrländer, U. (1986) *Die 'neue' Ausländerpolitik in Europa. Erfahrungen in den Aufnahme – und Entsendeländern*, Bonn: Verlag Neue Gesellschaft.

Krusell, I. (1980) 'Europol: Arbeitshypothese für eine kommende europäische Kriminalpolizeizusammenarbeit', in Bund Deutscher Kriminalbeambter (Hrsgb) *Grenzüberschreitende Verbrechenbekampfung im Spiegelbild Zwischenstaatlicher Verträge und gesetzlicher Regelungen*, Aachen.

Kube, E. (1986) *Systematische Kriminalprävention: ein strategisches Konzept mit praktischen Beispielen*, Wiesbaden: Bundeskriminalamt.

Kudriawcew, W.I., Karpiec, I.I., and Korobiejnikow, B.W. (eds) (1985) *Kurs sowietskoj kriminologii: Priedmiet, mietodologia, priestupnost i jejo prícziny, priestupnik*, Moscow: Juridiczeskaja Litieratura.

Kuhn, A. (1987) 'Körperverletzung als Konflikt: Zwischenbericht 1987 zum Projekt Handschlag', unpublished interim report of the Handschlag Project, Reutlingen.

Kuhn, A. and Rössner, D. (1987) 'Konstruktive Tatverarbeitung im Jugendstrafrecht: "Handschlag" statt Urteil', *Zeitschrift für Rechtspolitik* 20: 267–70.

Kuzniecowa, N.F. (1976) 'Umocnienie socjalistycznej praworzadnosci i organizacja walki z prezestepczoscia w swietle uchwal XXIV Zjazdu KPZR', in B. Holyst (ed.) *Kryminologia w krajach socjalistycznych*, Warszawa: Wydawnictwo Prawnicze.

Lab, S.P. (1988) *Crime Prevention: Approaches, Practices and Evaluations*, Cincinnati, OH: C.J. Anderson.

La Documentation Française (1987) *Aspects de la criminalité et de la délinquance constitués en France en 1986*, Paris: Ministry of Justice.

Lammich, S. and Nagy, F. (1985) 'Kriminalitätsentwicklung und Strafpraxis in Ungarn nach dem Inkrafttreten des StGB von 1978', *Monatsschrift für Strafrechtsreform und Kriminologie* 68: 176–86.

Landeskriminalamt Nordrhein-Westfalien (1987) *Polizeiliche Kriminalstatistik 1986*, Düsseldorf: Landeskriminalamt.

Langlais, S. (1974) *Polizeiliche Zusammenarbeit in Europa und die Rolle der IKPO*, in Bund Deutscher Kriminalbeamter (Hrsgb), pp. 50–7.

Larner, C. (1981) *Enemies of God*, London: Chatto & Windus.

Law and Contemporary Problems (1987) *Extraterritoriality of Economic Legislation*, special issue of *Law and Contemporary Problems* 50, 3.

Law Commission (1989) *Criminal Law Jurisdiction over Offences of Fraud and Dishonesty with a Foreign Element*, London: HMSO.

Leigh, L. (ed.) (1980) *Economic Crime in Europe*, London: Macmillan.

—— (1982) *The Control of Commercial Fraud*, Aldershot: Gower.

—— (1984) 'Shortcomings of the law concerning company frauds: the French response to the problem', *Company Lawyer* 5, 1: 35–9.

—— (1988) 'Territorial jurisdiction and fraud', Criminal Law Review, 280–9.

Leigh, L. and Smith A. (forthcoming) *Fraud in Europe: Towards 1992*, London: Blackstone Press.

Lekschas, J., Harrland, H., Hartmann, R., and Lehmann, G. (1983) *Kriminologie. Theoretische Grundlagen und Analysen*, Berlin: Staatsverlag der Deutschen Demokratischen Republik.

Levi, M. (1987a) *Regulating Fraud: White-Collar Crime and the Criminal Process*, London: Routledge.

—— (1987b) 'Crisis? What crisis? Reactions to commercial fraud in the United Kingdom', *Contemporary Crises* 11, 3: 207–21.

—— (forthcoming) *Customer Confidentiality, Money-Laundering, and Police–Bank Relationships: English Law and Practice in a Global Environment*, London: Chartered Institute of Bankers.

Levi, M. and Suddle, M. (1989) 'White-collar crime, shamelessness, and disintegration: the control of tax evasion in Pakistan', *Journal of Law and Society*, 4.

Lewis, R. (1989) 'European markets in cocaine', *Contemporary Crises* 13: 35–52.

Littas, R. (1979) 'The Sepat-Plan and its development', *International Criminal Police Review* 34, 327: 101–4.

L'Organisation Internationale de Police Criminelle – Interpol (1978) *Revue Internationale de Politique Criminelle* 34: 97–101.

Los, M. (1989) *The Second Economy in Marxist States*, Basingstoke: Macmillan.

McDermott, K. and King, R.D. (1988) 'Mind games: where the action is in prisons', *British Journal of Criminology* 28, 3: 357–77.

McIntosh, M. (1975) *The Organisation of Crime*, London: Macmillan.

Mack, J. (1975) *The Crime Industry*, London: Saxon House.

McCleod, E. (1982) *Women Working: Prostitution Now*, London: Croom Helm.

Magnusson, D. (ed.) (1985) *Economic Crime – Programs for Future Research*, Stockholm: National Council for Crime Prevention, Sweden.

Maguire, M. and Vagg, J. (1984) *The Watchdog Role of Boards of Visitors*, London: Home Office.

Maguire, M., Vagg, J., and Morgan, R. (eds) (1985) *Accountability and Prisons: Opening up a Closed World*, London: Tavistock.

Malewska-Peyre, H. (1982) *Crise d'identité et deviance chez les jeunes immigrants*, Vaucresson: La Documentation Française.

Mandaraka-Sheppard, A. (1986) *The Dynamics of Aggression in Women's Prisons in England*, Aldershot: Gower.

Mannheim, H. (1965) *Comparative Criminology*, London: Routledge & Kegan Paul.

Mansel, J. (1986) 'Die unterschiedliche Selektion von jungen Deutschen, Türken und Italienern auf dem Weg vom polizeilich Tatverdächtigen zum gerichtlich Verurteilten', *Monatsschrift für Kriminologie und Strafrechtsreform* 69: 309–25.

—— (1989) *Die Selektion der Organe der Strafrechtspflege am Beispiel von jungen Deutschen, Türken und Italienern*, Frankfurt/Berne/New York/Paris: Peter Lang Verlag.

Mayhew, P. (1984) 'Target-hardening: how much of an answer?' in R.

Clarke and T. Hope (eds) *Coping with Burglary: Research Perspectives on Policy*, Boston, Mass: Kluwer/Nijhoff.
Mayhew, P., Clarke, R.V.G., Sturman, A., and Hough, J.M. (1976) *Crime as Opportunity*, London: HMSO.
Mayhew, P., Elliott, D., and Dowds, L. (1989) *The 1988 British Crime Survey*, London: HMSO.
Menard, M. and Meurs, D. (1984) *Les Aggressions commises par les détenus contre les membres du personnel dans les établissements penitentiaires de la metropole 1982–1983*, Travaux et Documents no. 26, Paris: Ministère de la Justice/Direction de l'Administration Penitentiaire, Service des Etudes, de la Documentation et des Statistiques.
Middendorf, W. and Middendorf, D. (1984) 'Changing patterns of female criminality in Germany', in F. Adler (ed.) *The Incidence of Female Criminality in the Contemporary World*, New York: New York University Press.
Miethe, T. (1984) 'Types of consensus in public evaluations of crime: an illustration of strategies for measuring consensus', *Journal of Criminal Law and Criminology* 75: 459–73.
Minderheden Bulletin (1984) *Pers.-Documentatie beleid minderheden, afdeling voorlichting*, 's-Gravenhage: Ministerie Binnenlands Zaken.
Ministère de la Justice (1986) *Direction de l'Administration Penitentiaire: Rapport General sur l'Exercice 1985*, Paris: Ministère de la Justice.
—— (1987) *Direction de l'Administration Penitentiaire: Rapport General sur l'Exercice 1986*, Paris: Ministère de la Justice.
Ministerie van Justitie (n.d.) 'Extract from the prison regulations and other regulations governing the prison system: applicable to prisoners in Houses of Detention', pamphlet, The Hague: Ministerie van Justitie.
Ministry of the Interior (1987) *La Documentation Française*, Paris: Ministry of the Interior.
Ministry of Justice (1984) *The Price of Prisons Compared*, The Hague: Ministry of Justice.
Ministry of Justice (1989), Paris.
Monjardet, D. (1988) 'Le maintien de l'ordre: technique et ideologie professionnelles des CRS', *Deviance et Societé* 12, 2: 101–26.
Moody, S. and Tombs, J. (1982) *Prosecution in the Public Interest*, Edinburgh: Scottish Academic Press.
Morgan, R. (1987) 'Police accountability: developing the local infrastructure', *British Journal of Criminology* 27, 1: 87–96.
Morgan, R. and Macfarlane, A. (1985) *After Tarrant: Advice for Boards of Visitors Regarding Assistance for Prisoners at Adjudications*, 2nd edn, London: Association of Members of Boards of Visitors.
Morgan, R., Maguire, M., and Vagg, J. (1985) 'Overhauling the prison disciplinary system: notes for readers of the Prior Committee's report', in M. Maguire, J. Vagg, and R. Morgan (eds) *Accountability and Prisons: Opening up a Closed World*, London: Tavistock.
Moxon, D. (ed.) (1985) *Managing Criminal Justice: A Collection of Papers*, London: HMSO.
Naffine, N. (1987) *Female Crime*, Sydney: Allen & Unwin.

Nepote, J. (1970) 'La coopération des autorités policières en matières penale dans les rapports intra-européens', in *Droit pénal européen*, Brussels: Presses Universitaires de Bruxelles.

Newburn, T. (1988) *The Use and Enforcement of Compensation Orders in the Magistrates' Court*, Home Office Research Study no. 102, London: HMSO.

Newman, O. (1972) *Defensible Space*, New York: Macmillan.

OECD (1989) *Explanatory Report on the Convention of Mutual Administrative Assistance in Tax Matters*, Strasbourg: Council of Europe.

Oppermann, A. (1986) *Die Kriminalität junger Ausländer – Selektion oder soziale Mängellage*, Freiburg: Evangelische Fachhochschule für Sozialarbeit.

Orie, A.M.M. (1983) 'De verdachte tussen wal en schip of de systeembreuk in de kleine rechtshulp' in *Bij deze stand van zaken: bundel opstellen aangeboden aan A.L. Melai*, Arnhem: Gouda Quint.

Oriechow, W.W. (1976) 'O przyczynach przestepczości w spoleczenstiwie socjalistycznym', in B. Holyst (ed.) *Kryminologia w krajach socjalistycznych*, Warsaw: Wydawnictwo Prawnicze.

Osborough, N. (1975) *Borstal in Ireland*, Dublin: Institute of Public Administration.

Pease, K. (1984) 'Crime, race and reporting to the police', unpublished manuscript, University of Manchester.

Pelikan, C. (1987) 'Willige und unwillige Opfer', *Kriminalsoziologische Bibliographie* 14: 91–110.

Pelikan, C. and Pilgram, A. (1988) 'Die "Erfolgs-statistik" des Modellversuchs', *Kriminalsoziologische Bibliographie* 15: 55–79.

Petersilia, J. (1985) 'Racial disparities in the criminal justice system: a summary', *Crime and Delinquency* 31: 15–34.

Petrie, G. (1971) *A Singular Iniquity: The Campaigns of Josephine Butler*, London: Macmillan.

Pfeiffer, Ch. (1988) *Die Anordnung von Untersuchungshaft gegenüber 14–15 jährigen bzw. 14–21 jährigen in den 93 Landgerichtsbezirken der Bundesrepublik Deutschland*, Hanover: Kriminologisches Forschungsinstitut Niedersachsen.

Pilgram, A.(1987) *Phasen der Kriminaliserungspolitik in Österreich*, Vienna: Institute für Rechts und Kriminal-Soziologie.

Pitsela, A. (1986) *Straffälligkeit und kriminelle Viktimisierung ausländischer Minderheiten in der BRD*, Freiburg: Max-Planck-Institute.

Plenel, E. (1986) 'Police et terrorisme', *Esprit* 12: 7–20.

Plenska, E. (1984) 'Female crime in Poland', in F. Adler (ed.) *Incidence of Female Criminality in the Contemporary World*, New York: New York University Press.

POA (1984) *The Prison Disciplinary System: Submission to the Home Office Departmental Committee on the Prison Disciplinary System*, London: Prison Officers' Association.

Police Review (1989a) 'Hurd proposes European drugs unit', *Police Review* 28 April: 846.

—— (1989b) 'Germany to seize dealer's profits', *Police Review* 28 July: 1,509.

—— (1989c) 'Swiss drugs experiment leads to rise in crime', *Police Review* 18 August: 1,656.

—— (1989d) 'Lockerbie rift denied', *Police Review*, 3 November: 2,212.

Prison Department (n.d.) Personal communication.

Quinn, P. (1985) 'Prison management and prison discipline: a case study of change', in M. Maguire, J. Vagg, and R. Morgan (eds) *Accountability and Prisons: Opening up a Closed World*, London: Tavistock.

Reali, M. and Shapland, J. (1986) 'Breaking down barriers: the work of the community mental health service of Trieste in the prison and judicial settings', *International Journal of Law and Psychiatry* 8: 395–412.

Rebscher, E. (1981) *Rechtliche und organisatorische Grundlagen der internationalen Zusammenarbeit bei der Drogenbekämpfung*, Wiesbaden: Bundeskriminalamt.

Research Triangle Institute (1976) *Drug Use and Crime*, Research Triangle Park, NC: Research Triangle Institute.

Reuter, P. (1983) *Disorganised Crime: Illegal Markets and the Mafia*, Cambridge, Mass: MIT Press.

Richardson, G. (1985) 'Judicial intervention in prison life', in M. Maguire, J. Vagg, and R. Morgan (eds) *Accountability and Prisons: Opening up a Closed World*, London: Tavistock.

Rigaux, F. (1985) 'L'exercice de la justice répressive', *Annales de Droit de Louvain* 45, 1: 23–50.

Rock, P. (ed.) (1988a) *A History of British Criminology, British Journal of Criminology*, 28, 2.

—— (1988b) 'Governments, victims and policies in two countries', *British Journal of Criminology* 28, 1: 44–66.

Rosenbaum, D.P. (1988) 'Community crime prevention: a review and synthesis of the literature', *Justice Quarterly* 5, 3: 323–95.

Sack, F. and Steinert, H. (1984) *Protest und Reaktion*, Opladen: Westdeutscher Verlag.

Salewsky, F. (1974) 'Die Rauschgiftkriminalität und ihre Bekämpfung', in Bund Deutscher Kriminalbeamter *Europäische Gemeinschaft – auch für die Kriminalpolizei? Berichtsheft zur zweiten Fachtagung 'Kripo International 74'*, Berlin.

Savormin Lohman, P.M. and van Dijk, A.G. (1988) 'Neighbourhood watch in the Netherlands: the lessons of six projects', The Hague: National Crime Prevention Bureau.

Schaarschmidt, R. (1988) 'Methodische Anmerkungen zur Diskussion um die Kriminalitätsursachen im Sozialismus', in U. Ewald (ed.) *Gesellschafts theorie und Sozialwissenschaft in Kriminologie und Strafrechtswissenschaft. Ideen und Probleme*, Berlin. Kindler.

Schmid, A.P. (1983) *Political Terrorism: A Research Guide to Concepts, Theories, Data Bases and Literature*, Leiden: Rijksuniversiteit te Leiden.

Schmitz, C. and Hassebrauch, M. (1987) *Kurzinformation über den Braunschweiger Modellversuch 'Täter-Opfer-Ausgleich'*, Hanover: Criminological Research Institute of Lower Saxony.

Schneider, H.J. (1987) *Kriminologie*, Berlin/New York: Walter de Gruyter.

Schoutheete, Ph. de (1980) *La cooperation politique européene*, Brussels: Editions Labor.

Schreckling, J. (1989) 'Ausgleichsverläufe und – ergebnisse bei der "Waage"-Köln', paper given at the conference 'Täter-Opfer-Ausgleich – Zwischenbilanz und Perspektiven', Bonn.

Schwitters, B. (1978) *Dossier Interpol: de verborgen wereld van Interpol*, Amsterdam: Loeb and Van der Velden.

Scull, A. (1984) *Decarceration* (2nd edn), Cambridge: Polity.

Seifried, H. (1981) 'Deutsch-französische Zusammenarbiet bei der Verbrechensbekämpfung, *Kriminalistik* 35, 4: 169–73; Euregio Meuse-Rhin.

Sessar, K. (1981) *Rechtliche und soziale Prozesse einer Definition der Tötungskriminalität*, Freiburg: Max-Planck-Institute.

—— (1982) 'Offender retribution as part of a future criminal policy?', paper given to 4th International Symposium on Victimology, Tokyo, Japan.

Shapland, J. and Hobbs, D. (1989) 'Looking at policing', in R. Hood (ed.) *Crime and Criminal Policy in Europe*, Oxford: Centre for Criminological Research, University of Oxford.

Shapland, J. and Vagg, J. (1988) *Policing by the Public*, London: Routledge.

Shapland, J. and Wiles, P. (eds) (1989) *Business and Crime: A Consultation*, Swindon: Crime Concern.

Shapland, J., Willmore, J., and Duff, P. (1985) *Victims in the Criminal Justice System*, Aldershot: Gower.

Sheridan, M. (1989) 'Alarmed bankers impose checks on Mafia's loot', *The Independent*, 20 May.

Siemann, W. (1985) *Deutschlands Ruhe, Sicherheit und Ordnung: die Anfänge der politischen Polizei, 1806–1866*, Tübingen: Max Niemeyer Verlag.

Simon, R.J. (1975) *Women and Crime*, Toronto/London: Lexington Books.

Smart, C. (1977) *Women, Crime, and Criminology: A Feminist Critique*, London: Routledge & Kegan Paul.

—— (1979) 'The new female criminal: reality or myth?', *British Journal of Criminology* 19, 1: 50–9.

Smart, C. and Smart, B. (1979) *Women, Sexuality and Social Control*, London: Routledge & Kegan Paul.

Smith, D.J. and Gray, J. (1983) *Police and People in London*, vol. IV, London: The Police in Action, PSI.

Smith, L. (1988) 'Images of women – decision-making in the courts', in A. Morris and C. Wilkinson (eds) *Women and the Penal System*, Cropwood Papers no. 19, Cambridge: Cambridge Institute of Criminology.

Sprott, W., Jephcott, A., and Carter, M. (1954) *The Social Background of Delinquency*, Nottingham: University of Nottingham.

Stanko, E. (1984) *Intimate Intrusions*, London: Routledge & Kegan Paul.

Staudt, G. (1983) *Kriminelles und konformes Verhalten der Gastarbeiternachkommen*, Saarbrücken: University of Saarbrücken.

Steffen, W. (1983) *Intensität und Perseveranz krimineller Verhaltensweisen*, Munich: Bayerisches Landeskriminalamt.

Steiner, J. (1988) *Textbook on EEC Law*, London: Blackstone Press.

Steinhilper, U. (1986) *Definitions – und Entscheidungsprozesse bei sexuell motivierten Gewaltdelikten*, Constance, Switzerland: Universitätsverlag.

Stevens, P. and Willis, C. (1979) *Race, Crime and Arrests*, London: HMSO.
Stevens, P. and Willis, C. (1981) *Ethnic Minorities and Complaints Against the Police*, London: HMSO.
Stimson, G., Aldritt, L., Dolan, K., Donahoe, M., and Lart, R. (1988) *Injecting Equipment Exchange Schemes: Final Report*, London: Monitoring Research Group, Goldsmiths' College, University of London.
Strobl, Killius, and Vorbrugg (1986) *Business Law Guide to Germany*, London: CCH.
Sutherland, E.H. (1983) *White-Collar Crime*, London: Yale University Press.
Swan, D. (1988) *The Economics of the Common Market*, 6th edn, Harmondsworth: Penguin.
Swart, A.H.J. (1984) *Internationalisering van de strafrechtspleging*, in C. Kelk, P. Moediko, M. Moerings, and A.H.J. Swart (eds) *Grenzen en mogelijkheden; opstellen over en rondom de strafrechtspleging*, Nijmegen: Ars Aequi Libri.
Swigert, V. and Farrell, R. (1981) 'Corporate homicide: definitional processes in the construction of deviance', *Law and Society Review*, 15: 161–82.
Taylor, I., Walton, P. and Young, J. (1973) *The New Criminology*, London: Routledge & Kegan Paul.
Tiedemann, K. (1980) 'Antitrust law and criminal policy in Western Europe', in L. Leigh (ed.) *Economic Crime in Europe*, London: Macmillan.
Tuck, M. and Southgate, P. (1981) *Ethnic Minorities and Policing: A Survey of the Experience of West Indians and Whites*, London: HMSO.
Tutt, N. (1989) *Europe on the Fiddle*, London: Christopher Helm.
Tweede Kamer (1986–7) 20 031, nos 1-2. See the 'Notitie Grensbewaking' that was submitted by the Dutch government to the Dutch Parliament in July 1987.
Unnever, J.D. and Hembroff, L.A. (1988) 'The prediction of racial/ethnic sentencing disparities: an expectation states approach', *Journal of Research in Crime and Delinquency* 25: 53–82.
UNSDRI (1988) *Informal Mechanisms of Crime Control*, Rome: United Nations Social Defence Institute.
Vagg, J. and Vossen, R. (1988) 'Accountability and prisons: some European comparisons', paper to the 10th International Congress on Criminology, Hamburg, 4–9 September.
Vagó, T. (1976) 'Niektóre poglady kryminologii socjalistycznej dotyczace przyczyn przestepczosci', in B. Holyst (ed.) *Kriminologia w krajach socjalistycznych*, Warsaw: Wydawnictwo Prawnicze.
Van Dijk, J.J.M. (1988a) 'Victim rights: a right to better services or a right to active participation', in J. van Dijk, C. Haffmans, F. Ruter, J. Schutte, and S. Stolwijk (eds) *Criminal Law in Action*, Arnhem: Gouda Quint.
—— (1988b) 'Institutionalisierte Kriminalprävention: eine kritische Bewertung von Modellen in Europa', in *Kriminalitaetsbekämpfung als Gesamtgesellschaftliche Aufgabe*, Wiesbaden: Bundeskriminalamt.
—— (1989) 'Crime prevention: current state and prospects', in *Proceedings II European Colloquium on Crime and Public Policy in Europe*, Freiburg: Max-Planck-Institut.

Van Dijk, J.J.M. and Junger-Tas, J. (1988) 'Trends in crime prevention in the Netherlands', in T. Hope and M. Shaw (eds) *Communities and Crime Reduction*, London: HMSO.

Van Dijk, J.J.M., Mayhew, P., and Killias, M. (1990) *Experiences with Crime Across the World: Results of the 1989 International Telephone Survey*, The Hague: Kluwer.

Van Soomeren, P. (1989) 'Business and crime: a foreigner's view', in J. Shapland and P. Wiles (eds) *Business and Crime: A Consultation*, Swindon: Crime Concern.

Van Vliet, H. (1989) 'Drug policy as a management strategy', *International Journal on Drug Policy* 1, 1: 27–9.

Viet, F. (1989) 'Erfahrungen mit TOA in der JGH Braunschweig nach Empfehlung durch Polizeibeamte', paper given at the conference 'Täter-Opfer-Ausgleich – Zwischenbilanz und Perspektiven', Bonn.

Villmow, B. (1983) 'Kriminalität der jungen Ausländer: Ausmaß und Struktur des abweichenden Verhaltens und gesellschaftlicher Reaktion', in H.-J. Kerner, H. Goppinger, and F. Streng (eds) *Kriminologie – Psychiatrie – Strafrecht*, Heidelberg: Beck.

—— (1984) 'Implications of research on victimisation for criminal and social policy', *European Committee on Crime Problems*, Strasbourg: Council of Europe.

—— (1985) 'Gastarbeiterkriminalität', in G. Kaiser, H.-J. Kerner, F. Sack, and H. Schellhoss (eds) *Kleines Kriminologisches Wörterbuch*, Heidelberg: C.F. Müller.

—— (1989) 'Reaktionen von Polizei und Justiz auf Ausländer-delinquenz', in Bundeskriminalamt (ed.) *Ausländerkriminalität in der Bundes- republik Deutschland*, Wiesbaden: Bundeskriminalamt.

Vodopivec, K. (1981) 'Vergleichende Kriminologie: Jugoslavien', in H.J. Schneider (ed.) *Die Psychologie des 20. Jahrhunderts. Band XIV. Auswirkungen auf die Kriminologie*, Zürich: Kindler.

Walker, M.A. (1988) 'The court disposal of young males, by race, in London in 1983', *British Journal of Criminology* 28, 4: 441–60.

Wallace, W. (1989) 'Sans Frontières', *Guardian*, 6 January.

Waller, I. (1989) 'Current trends in crime prevention in Europe: implications for Canada', Ottawa: Department of Justice.

Walter, I. (1989) *Secret Money*, 2nd edn, London: Unwin Hyman.

Walter, M. (1987) Kriminalität junger Ausländer – Forschungstand und Offene Fragen – Bewährungshilfe.

Waters, R. (1988) 'Race and the criminal justice process: two empirical studies on social inquiry reports and ethnic minority defendants', *British Journal of Criminology* 28, 1: 82–94.

Weijden, H. van der (1986) 'Interpol: coördinerend steunpunt in wereldwijde politiesamenweerking of postkantoor', *Tap* 40, 4: 13–16.

Wells, C. (1988) 'The decline and rise of English murder: corporate crime and individual responsibility', *Criminal Law Review*, June: 788–801.

Werdenich, W. (1988) 'Die Täter – die Opfer – die Betreuer. Aus der Supervision einer neuen Form der Sozialarbeit', *Kriminalsoziologische Bibliographie* 15: 135–44.

Wijngaart, Ch. van der (1980) 'Euroterrorisme en "espace judiciaire européen": de fundamentele rechten van het individu in het gedrang?', *Rechtskundig Weekblad* 43, 40: 2,675–93.

Wiles, P. (1989) 'Ethnic minorities, crime and public policy', in R. Hood (ed.) *Crime and Criminal Policy in Europe*, Oxford: Centre for Criminological Research, University of Oxford.

Wilkins, L. (1984) *Consumerist Criminology*, Aldershot: Gower.

Williams, J., Dunning, E., and Murphy, P. (1989) *Hooligans Abroad*, London: Routledge.

Wilson, J.Q. (1975) *Thinking about Crime*, New York: Basic Books.

Winkel, F. (1987) 'Response generalisation in crime prevention campaigns', *British Journal of Criminology* 27, 2: 155–73.

With, J. (1984) 'Criminality among Black people in the Bijlmermeer', in J. Brown (ed.) *Policing and Social Policy*, London: Police Review Publishing.

Wood, J. (1989) 'The serious fraud office', *Criminal Law Review* March: 175–84.

World Health Organization (1984) *World Health Statistics Annual*, Geneva: World Health Organization.

Young, J. (1988) 'Recent developments in criminology', in M. Haralambos (ed.) *Developments in Sociology*, vol. IV, London: Causeway.

Zauberman R. (1985) 'Les victimes: etude du crime ou sociologie du penal?', *L'Année Sociologique* XXV: 31–59.

—— (1989) 'Victim-related alternatives to the criminal justice system: compensation, restitution and mediation – some comments on Martin Killias' paper', paper given to the II European Colloquium on Crime and Public Policy in Europe, to be published by the Max-Planck-Institute.

Zellick, G. (1981) 'The prison rules and the courts', *Criminal Law Review*: 602.

—— (1982) 'The prison rules and the courts: a postscript', *Criminal Law Review*: 575.

Zwirbul, W.K. (1976) 'Spoleczno-hystoryczny aspekt badania przychzyn przestepczosci', in B. Holyst (ed.) *Kryminologia w krajach socjalistycznych*, Warsaw: Wydawnictwo Prawnicze.

Name index

Subject index